CONTENTS

Environmental Health Criteria 51

GUIDE TO SHORT-TERM TESTS FOR DETECTING MUTAGENIC AND CARCINOGENIC CHEMICALS

Prepared for the IPCS by the International Commission for Protection Against Environmental Mutagens and Carcinogens

Published under the joint sponsorship of
the United Nations Environment Programme,
the International Labour Organisation,
and the World Health Organization

World Health Organization
Geneva, 1985

The **International Programme on Chemical Safety (IPCS)** is a joint venture of the United Nations Environment Programme, the International Labour Organisation, and the World Health Organization. The main objective of the IPCS is to carry out and disseminate evaluations of the effects of chemicals on human health and the quality of the environment. Supporting activities include the development of epidemiological, experimental laboratory, and risk-assessment methods that could produce internationally comparable results, and the development of manpower in the field of toxicology. Other activities carried out by IPCS include the development of know-how for coping with chemical accidents, coordination of laboratory testing and epidemiological studies, and promotion of research on the mechanisms of the biological action of chemicals.

ISBN 92 4 154191 1

PRINTED IN FINLAND
85/5761 — VAMMALA — 5500

NOTE TO READERS OF THE CRITERIA DOCUMENTS

Every effort has been made to present information in the criteria documents as accurately as possible without unduly delaying their publication. In the interest of all users of the environmental health criteria documents, readers are kindly requested to communicate any errors that may have occurred to the Manager of the International Programme on Chemical Safety, World Health Organization, Geneva, Switzerland, in order that they may be included in corrigenda, which will appear in subsequent volumes.

*   *   *

A detailed data profile and a legal file can be obtained from the International Register of Potentially Toxic Chemicals, Palais des Nations, 1211 Geneva 10, Switzerland (Telephone no. 988400 - 985850).

CONTRIBUTORS

The following experts participated in the preparation of this document:

Dr I.-D. Adler, Institute for Genetics, GSF, Neuherberg, Federal Republic of Germany

Dr J. Cole, MRC Cell Mutation Unit, University of Sussex, Brighton, Sussex, United Kingdom

Dr N. Danford, University College of Swansea, Swansea, United Kingdom

Dr U. Ehling, Institute for Genetics, GSF, Neuherberg, Federal Republic of Germany

Dr M. Parry, Genetics Department, University College of Swansea, Swansea, United Kingdom

Dr R. Roderick, Sittingbourne Research Centre, Sittingbourne, Kent, United Kingdom

Dr S. Venitt, Chester Beatty Research Institute, Institute for Cancer Research, Royal Cancer Hospital, Pollards Wood Research Station, Chalfont St. Giles, Buckinghamshire, United Kingdom

Dr W. Vogel, Department of Radiation Genetics and Chemical Mutagenesis, Sylvius Laboratories, Leiden, The Netherlands

Dr R. Waters, Genetics Department, University College of Swansea, Swansea, United Kingdom

PREAMBLE

During the past few years, great advances have been made in understanding the processes leading to malignant disease. It is clear that alterations in genetic material are involved in these processes and that a great many carcinogens are capable of inducing such alterations under appropriate conditions. Heritable alterations in germ cells may also be induced by certain chemicals and may constitute a genetic risk. Numerous short-term tests have been developed to detect the ability of chemicals to cause such changes and are being used routinely and successfully, on a large scale. There is a widespread desire to evaluate the data obtained from short-term tests and to generate such data in areas of the world where the necessary combinations of expertise may not yet be available.

The International Commission for Protection Against Environmental Mutagens and Carcinogens (ICPEMC), an assembly of scientists with expertise in the fields of environmental mutagenesis, carcinogenesis, genetic toxicology, and epidemiology, was therefore pleased to respond to the request of the International Programme on Chemical Safety of the World Health Organization, to prepare a document containing guidance in the field of short-term testing for mutagens and carcinogens with genetic activity. This document represents the views of ICPEMC and is published by IPCS in an attempt to stimulate scientific discussion, as well as to provide guidance on the use of genotoxicity tests in chemical safety programmes. Although short-term tests to screen for mutagenicity and carcinogenicity are useful, they have their difficulties and limitations. For example, while the majority of chemical initiators of carcinogenesis give positive results in tests for genetic change, it is not necessarily true that all chemicals with genetic activity are carcinogens. Moreover, there are carcinogens and cocarcinogens that are not readily detected by mutagenicity tests and that may act by mechanisms of quite a different nature. Such substances are necessarily excluded from consideration here, but that does not mean that they may not be of the same importance. There are differences of approach in genetic toxicology, as in most other branches of science. The present document reflects a widely-used approach that may be regarded as good contemporary practice. It should be emphasized that it does not claim to be definitive or to contain recommendations for regulatory action either in connection with the kind or number of tests that should be carried out, or the regulatory decisions that may be taken on the basis of the results of such tests. It is designed to explain the types of test that are commonly employed and the meaning that the results of such tests may have in the assessment of possible human hazard, as far as is possible with current scientific knowledge.

It is obvious that any assessment of test results in terms of mutagenic or genotoxic hazard can be properly made only in the context of the whole toxicological profile of a substance and its use. ICPEMC is currently working towards a position with regard to the selection of short-term tests and its recommendations should be available in the near future.

Current practice is still rapidly evolving and should not be considered as fixed. Moreover, what might be considered feasible in scientifically advanced countries with large resources of expertise might be quite inappropriate in developing countries. The latter, however, provide the raison d'être of the present document, which is offered in a spirit of helpfulness in the hope that it may enable short-term genotoxicity tests to be used in a reasonable manner.

1. INTRODUCTION

It has been known for many years that some chemicals can cause cancer in man. More recently, there has been a growing awareness of the possibility that chemicals may also produce mutations in human germ cells thus influencing the frequency of genetic or heritable diseases. Many thousands of chemicals, including pharmaceutical products, domestic and food chemicals, pesticides, and petroleum products are present in the environment and new chemicals are being introduced each year. In addition, there are many compounds that occur naturally, which are known to be mutagenic and/or carcinogenic (e.g., mycotoxins in foods). It is important, therefore, that chemicals to which people are exposed, either intentionally (e.g., therapeutically), in the course of their daily life (e.g., in domestic products, cosmetics, etc.), or inadvertently (e.g., in pesticides) are tested for their potential to produce cancer and genetic damage (mutations).

A few chemicals have been identified as carcinogenic because of their known association with cancer in man. However, carcinogenic activity is usually determined by the ability of a chemical to produce tumours during the life-time exposure of laboratory animals. Studies of this kind may last for two or three years and require the use of scarce resources and expertise. This has led to the search for alternative ways of detecting chemicals with cancer-producing potential and a number of relatively inexpensive assays have been developed, many using biological systems rather than whole mammals. Because such assay systems need far less time to complete than classical long-term studies in rodents they are referred to as "short-term tests".

Although the results of epidemiological studies have confirmed that exposure to a number of chemicals, such as vinyl chloride and beta-naphthylamine, can cause cancer in man, convincing epidemiological evidence that chemicals constitute a mutagenic hazard for man is not yet available. It is known that genetic defects cause a significant proportion of human diseases, but the contribution of environmental chemicals to genetic disease is unknown. This is not surprising as the possibility of such a danger to health has only been apparent for about one generation.

The information that determines the characteristics of a cell or organism is contained in the genetic material of the cell, which is composed of deoxyribonucleic acid (DNA). DNA is composed of sub-units of deoxyribonucleotides, which themselves consist of a pentose sugar (2-deoxyribose), a phosphate ester, and a purine or pyrimidine nitrogenous base. These sub-units form a 3-dimensional helical double-stranded

structure (Watson & Crick, 1953). Each of the two strands
consists of a linear array of the deoxyribose sugar molecules
linked together in a chain by phosphate molecules. The
strands are joined side-by-side by hydrogen bonds between
complementary pairs of the purine and pyrimidine bases. The
complementary pairs of bases are guanine (a purine) paired
with cytosine (a pyrimidine) and adenine (a purine) paired
with thymine (a pyrimidine). The unique sequence of bases,
taken in groups of three, or triplets, forms the genetic code,
each triplet coding for a particular amino acid. Sequences of
triplets provide uniquely the information necessary for the
synthesis of a functional protein or enzyme. Such a
functional sequence of bases is known as a gene. Genetic
information is passed from one cell generation to the next by
precise duplication of the strands and equal distribution of
the DNA, prior to cell division (i.e., the mitosis of somatic
cells or the meiosis of germ cells) and is responsible for the
faithful handing on of all the characteristics of one
generation to the next generation. This fundamental genetic
process is common to all organisms ranging from a simple
bacterial cell to a complex mammal or plant. In higher
organisms, the long strands of DNA are bound to proteins
(histones) and are organised into a number of complex
structures called chromosomes, located in the nucleus of the
cell.

With the exception of the germ cells, which carry a single
set of chromosomes and are termed haploid, the cells of higher
organisms contain duplicate sets of chromosomes, one set
derived from each parent, i.e., they are diploid.

Diploid cells, therefore, carry a pair of each of the
functional genes, which occupy a precise position or locus
along the length of the DNA of a particular chromosome. The
paired genes may be identical (homozygous) or functionally
different (heterozygous); heterozygous forms of the same gene
are called alleles. In many cases, one of the two alleles has
a dominant function over its partner. Such partners are
called dominant (or partially dominant) and recessive (or
partially recessive). Occasionally, a pair of alleles are
expressed independently of each other and are regarded as
co-dominant.

Genes carried by the X-chromosome behave differently. As
males have only one X-chromosome, the genes are not carried in
pairs and a gene on this chromosome is expressed as a dominant
or recessive X-linked characteristic. Although females have
two X-chromosomes, a similar, though more complex situation
exists, as only one of the two X-chromosomes expresses its
genes in a particular cell type. The fact that the basic
helical structure of DNA and the genetic coding is common to
all living organisms, whether they are bacteria, plants, or

mammals, means that data obtained from studies of the effects of a chemical on one species can be used to predict the possible genetic response of another species to the same chemical.

Alterations to the information carried by the DNA occur as a result of small changes in the structure of the DNA molecule, whereby the base sequence transmitted to the next generation is changed, and this may result in descendants with different characteristics to the parent. The alterations are, in effect, mutations and, though many of them are detrimental, some mutations are compatible with a normal, healthy existence, being responsible for the subtle differences between members of a species and constituting the driving force of evolution.

Mutagenic chemicals interact with DNA causing changes in its structure. This may result in the loss, addition, or replacement of bases, thus altering their sequence in the DNA and affecting the fidelity of the genetic message.

The effect of these mutational changes may be to prevent the synthesis of functional proteins completely (i.e., inhibition of gene expression) or may lead to the synthesis of proteins with modified structure and enzymes with altered activity and specificity. Where mutations lead to changes in the genetic information carried by male or female germ cells, the progeny of such affected parents may express the mutation as some form of heritable abnormality or disease. When mutations occur in the somatic cells of a complex organism, they may produce irreversible changes in the cell that may ultimately be involved in producing a cancerous growth.

Mutation of one of a pair of genes may lead to a change in gene expression that can override the function of the normal partner and is called a dominant mutation. Recessive mutations are expressed only when both genes carry the same recessive mutation. For example, a recessive mutation inherited from the male parent will only be expressed in the progeny if the same recessive gene is also inherited from the female parent.

Cells can survive potentially lethal damage to the DNA, because of the activity of a series of enzyme-mediated processes that are generally termed DNA repair. The simplest form of DNA repair involves removal (excision) of the chemically-altered portion and the repair of the gap left in the DNA strand by the synthesis of new DNA using the undamaged sister strand as a template. Damage to DNA that is not repaired by this mechanism interferes with normal DNA synthesis (i.e., DNA replication). This stimulates another kind of DNA repair (post-replication repair) which, because it is not always accurate (i.e., it is error-prone), may lead to mutagenic changes in the DNA. The detection of unusual

excision DNA repair activity, so called unscheduled DNA
synthesis, in mammalian cells (as a response to damage to the
DNA) forms the basis of an important assay for identifying
chemicals that cause damage to DNA (section 2.3).

Damage to DNA may be expressed as mutations at the
chromosome level (i.e., chromosomal aberrations or chromosomal
mutations) or at the level of the gene (i.e., gene or point
mutations). Chromosomal mutations may be observed as changes
in the structure of the chromosome (structural aberrations) or
in the number of chromosomes in a cell (numerical aberrations
or aneuploidy). Structural aberrations are a consequence of
DNA damage while numerical changes are usually caused by
defects in the accurate distribution of chromosomes during
cell division, i.e., DNA damage may not be involved.

Mutations contribute significantly to human diseases and
congenital malformations, though the extent of this
contribution is not precisely known. Some diseases such as
Down's syndrome (Trisomy 21) are associated with structural or
numerical chromosomal abnormalities. Others are a result of
mutations of single genes and there are other diseases and
congenital abnormalities for which a genetic alteration may be
partly responsible. Sickle cell anaemia is a disease caused
by the inheritance of a single mutant gene that is responsible
for the synthesis of an abnormal haemoglobin molecule. In the
homozygous state, i.e., where the mutant gene is inherited
from both parents, the resulting disease is severe.
Heterozygous individuals carry only a single mutant gene and
suffer from the relatively mild sickle cell trait. Because of
the resistance of sickle cell red blood cells to the malarial
parasite, carriers of the trait have a selective advantage
over unaffected individuals and the mutant gene is maintained
at a high frequency in certain populations.

Although there is no definitive evidence that exposure to
chemicals is responsible for any of the known human genetic
disorders, experimental evidence from other mammals have shown
that chemicals can produce both chromosomal and gene mutations
of the type that are associated with human genetic diseases.
There is little direct evidence to suggest that man is any
less susceptible than other mammals to the effects of exposure
to mutagenic chemicals.

Alterations in the structure and function of DNA are
believed to play a crucial role in the production of cancer by
chemicals. Carcinogenesis is a multistage process that may
take years to evolve and a number of different factors
influence the progression from a normally functioning cell to
an invasive neoplastic tumour. (A carcinogen is defined as an
agent that significantly increases the frequency of malignant
neoplasms in a population; carcinogens may be physical,
chemical, or biological agents). The complex mechanisms by

which chemicals induce malignancy are not fully understood, but there is evidence that suggests the occurrence of four major stages following an adequate exposure of a mammal (including man) to a chemical carcinogen:

(a) transport of the chemical from the site of entry into the body and, in many cases, metabolic modification of the chemical (principally in the liver) to a more reactive form;

(b) interaction of the molecule or its reactive metabolite with the molecular target in the cell (the most important of which is DNA);

(c) expression of the DNA damage as a potentially carcinogenic lesion; and

(d) progression, influenced by modifying factor(s), and proliferation to form a malignant tumour.

Some carcinogenic chemicals appear to be responsible for only one part of the process and are not regarded as complete carcinogens. For example, many chemicals that interact with DNA and are thus mutagenic appear to initiate the process by inducing the primary DNA lesion. These are called initiators and the damage they cause is generally irreversible. Other compounds have been shown to influence the expression and progression of the initial DNA change and are called tumour enhancers. Some of these do not interact with DNA, they are not mutagenic and include the so-called tumour promoters. A third group includes chemicals known as complete carcinogens in that they are probably capable of both initiating and promoting activity. All chemicals that produce DNA damage leading to mutations or cancer, including initiators and complete carcinogens, are described as genotoxic.

The animal bioassay for detecting carcinogenic chemicals is a large, complex and very expensive scientific study using some hundreds of rodents to which the suspect chemical is administered for most of their life span. Similarly, the specific locus test in mice (Searle, 1975), which is one of the few currently available assays for detecting heritable gene mutations in mammals, requires the examination of many thousands of offspring and is equally expensive and time-consuming. Thus, of the multitude of chemicals introduced into the environment this century, and the hundreds of new compounds being synthesized each year, only a small fraction can be tested in conventional animal studies. For this reason, the last decade has seen the introduction of a number of relatively rapid tests for detecting mutagenic and

carcinogenic chemicals. Such tests are economical in
resources and produce results in a matter of weeks. Almost
all of these short-term procedures are based on the
demonstration of chromosomal damage, gene mutations, or DNA
damage, and many of them are in vitro assays (i.e., conducted
in experimental biological systems without the use of live
animals). As will be described in section 2, the test
organisms range from bacteria and yeasts to insects, plants,
and cultured animal cells and there are also short-term tests
in which laboratory animals are exposed to test chemicals for
periods of a few hours to, at most, a few weeks. In practice,
a suspect chemical is first tested using in vitro procedures,
to study its ability to react with DNA and thus induce
mutations. It may then be necessary to determine its
genotoxicity for intact animals by testing in short-term
mammalian (in vivo) assays.

The concept that carcinogenic chemicals cause cancer by a
mutagenic mechanism is the basis of the somatic mutation
theory of cancer induction. Between 1955 and 1970, there were
many attempts to demonstrate the mutagenicity of carcinogens
using simple bacterial assays but these experiments failed to
show a direct relationship between mutation and cancer.
Following the pioneering studies of Miller & Miller (1966), it
was realized that the majority of chemical carcinogens were
biologically inactive until they were enzymatically converted
into reactive molecules. Such chemicals are referred to as
pro-carcinogens. Intermediate metabolites that are the
precursors of the ultimate reactive molecule (i.e., the
molecule capable of reacting with DNA) are known as proximate
carcinogens. Cancer-inducing chemicals are often poorly
soluble in water and, like most foreign compounds entering an
organism, undergo a sequence of metabolic reactions intended
to detoxify them and if necessary convert them into more
water-soluble products, which can then be excreted by the
kidneys. In some cases, these metabolic reactions produce
carcinogenic chemicals, converting them into proximate and
ultimate carcinogenic metabolites. Most ultimate carcinogenic
molecules are electrophilic reactants capable of binding with
nucleophilic sites on DNA and other macromolecules (Miller &
Miller, 1971).

The major classes of chemical carcinogens are activated by
an oxidative reaction catalysed by microsomal mixed-function
oxidases, though other enzyme systems influence this
activation. Appropriate enzymes are present in most mammalian
tissues, the highest activity occurring in the liver. In
bacteria and most cultures of mammalian cells, mixed-function
oxidase activity is either absent or very low and they are
therefore not capable of activating the majority of
carcinogens at a significant rate. Insects have a complex

metabolic capability and appear to be capable of activating a wide range of pro-carcinogens. Yeast cells are also capable of limited foreign-compound metabolism. In the early 1970s, Garner et al. (1971) and Malling (1971), recognizing the significance of the metabolic activation of chemicals, devised experiments in which mammalian enzymes and bacterial cells were combined in a single assay. This led to the introduction of the first useful screening assay for carcinogenic chemicals, i.e., the Salmonella typhimurium reversion test described by Professor Bruce Ames and his colleagues (Ames et al., 1973). Essential aspects of mammalian metabolism are now introduced into many short-term in vitro assays by the incorporation of an enzyme-rich, cell-free extract of mammalian tissues. The most commonly used preparation is the post-mitochondrial supernatent (referred to as the "S9" fraction), obtained after high speed centrifugation of a homogenate of rat liver.

Although more than a hundred "test systems" for investigating genotoxicity have been described in the literature, ranging through the biological phyla from bacteriophage to mammals, less than 20 are in regular use and some of these are only available in specialised laboratories. The most widely-accepted systems are summarized below and described in detail in section 2.

Assays that involve the use of bacteria for detecting mutagenic chemicals are the most-extensively used and, in general, the most thoroughly validated. Unlike higher organisms, in which the DNA is organized into complex chromo-somal structures, bacteria contain a single circular molecule of DNA that is readily accessible to chemicals that can penetrate the cell wall. Bacterial tests also have the advantage that a population of many millions of cells with a relatively short generation time can be tested in a single assay. In the classical techniques, strains of bacteria are used that already contain mutations of specific genes. For example, a mutation at the histidine locus in S. typhimurium removes the ability of the bacterium to synthesize histidine and such mutants cannot survive in culture medium lacking this nutrient. Reversion at this locus enables the cell to synthesize histidine again and thus proliferate in medium lacking the amino acid. Mutations induced by test-chemicals, i.e., "reverse" mutations, are detected by the growth of the "revertant" bacteria to form colonies in appropriate selective culture media. Reverse mutation refers to reversion of an existing mutation, while forward mutation refers to the formation of a new mutation (section 2.1). Bacterial assays can be adapted for detecting mutagenic metabolites in body fluids (e.g., urine, blood, plasma) from exposed animals or human beings.

Yeast and fungi occupy a position between bacteria and animal cells in terms of genetic complexity. The structure of fungal DNA and its organisation into chromosomes is similar in many ways to that of mammals. Both haploid and diploid forms can be used in genetic assays. Tests using yeasts, such as Saccharomyces cerevisiae, are available for detecting both forward and reverse mutations and a variety of other genetic changes (section 2.2). Certain strains of yeast can be used to detect chemicals that induce aneuploidy (i.e., unequal distribution of chromosomes during cell division) and there is some evidence that non-genotoxic carcinogens can be identified using these strains.

The demonstration of DNA repair activity in mammalian cells is indirect evidence of DNA damage. DNA repair can be detected in a simple mammalian cell culture assay that involves the measurement of "repair" or "unscheduled" DNA synthesis (UDS) (section 2.3). The assay is based on the fact that thymidine is incorporated into DNA during both normal and repair synthesis. Cells treated with the suspect chemical are exposed to radioactive isotope-labelled (i.e., tritiated) thymidine at a stage when normal DNA synthesis is dormant or suppressed. The amount of radiolabelled thymidine detected in the DNA is a measure of DNA repair synthesis and, thus, an indication of primary DNA damage.

Chemicals can be tested for their ability to induce chromosomal damage either in mammals, insects, cultured mammalian cells, or in plants. Mammalian cell cultures provide a convenient test system and either established cell lines or human blood lymphocytes can be used (section 2.4). Analysis of metaphase chromosomes in cells from the bone marrow of rats, mice, or hamsters is a well-established technique for studying chromosome damage in vivo (section 2.8). Alternatively, chromosome fragments can be identified as micronuclei in certain bone marrow cells and in other tissues and the "micronucleus test" has proved to be a relatively simple assay for detecting chemicals capable of damaging chromosomes.

Cultures of mammalian cells can also be used to investigate the induction of gene mutations by chemicals (section 2.5). The principles involved are similar to those of microbial assays, i.e., cells are cultured in medium containing the suspect chemical and are then sub-cultured into a selective medium in which only mutant cells can survive. The number of cells that proliferate to form colonies is a measure of the number of cells that have undergone a forward mutation at the specific gene locus.

As described earlier in this section, bacteria, yeasts, and cultured mammalian cells may lack the enzymes necessary for the conversion of many carcinogens and mutagens to a molecular form that will react with DNA. Assays using these systems must, therefore, be supplemented with a suitable mammalian microsomal enzyme preparation. Many insects are able to activate a wide range of genotoxic chemicals and the demonstration of genetic changes in Drosophila melanogaster (the fruit fly) forms a useful assay for investigating carinogenic and mutagenic chemicals (section 2.7).

Because of the tremendous advances made in the use of microbial and mammalian cell procedures in genetic toxicology, plant material is less often used for studying mutagenic chemicals than previously. However, the use of plants such as the bean (Vicia faba), the onion (Allium cepa), the spiderwort (Tradescantia paludosa), maize (Zea mays), barley (Hordeum vulgare), and the soybean (Glycine max) may have significant advantages over other systems and their value in screening chemicals for mutagenic activity has still tu be fully explored (section 2.6). Investigation of genetic changes at both the gene and chromosomal level can be conducted in plants without the complicated laboratory facilities required for other types of assay and this may be a great advantage under certain circumstances. A possible disadvantage is that the metabolic pathways in plants differ in many respects from those in mammals. Thus, meaningful extrapolation to man of data obtained in plant studies is uncertain at present.

Data obtained from non-mammalian organisms and cultured mammalian cells determine whether a chemical or its metabolite(s) is capable of interacting with DNA and producing genetic damage. Two procedures are described in section 2 that are used to investigate the mutagenic activity of chemicals in the intact animal. The first (section 2.8) is designed to detect chromosome damage in the somatic cells of rodents. The second (section 2.9) is the dominant lethal assay that can identify chemicals capable of inducing genetic damage in the reproductive or germ cells of animals. In this test, male rats or mice are dosed with the suspect chemical and mated with untreated females. Certain types of chromosomal damage induced in the male germ cells are lethal to the fertilised ova and this can be detected by examination of the uterine contents.

Before short-term assays can be used to screen chemicals for potential carcinogenic activity with any degree of confidence, their sensitivity and accuracy for this purpose must be thoroughly validated. The first comprehensive validation of bacterial tests for detecting carcinogens was conducted by Ames and his colleagues (McCann et al., 1975) using a combination of bacteria (Salmonella) and mammalian microsomal enzymes. In this study, in which 300 chemicals were tested, approximately 90% of carcinogens were bacterial mutagens and 90% of non-carcinogens failed to show mutagenic activity. Following this, Purchase et al. (1978) investigated 120 carefully-selected chemicals in a series of six short-term tests. Again, the Ames bacterial mutation test gave a predictive value for carcinogenic potential of about 90%. Analyses of these and later studies showed that the success rate of mutagenicity tests for detecting carcinogens was influenced by the type or class of chemical selected for testing and the criteria on which the carcinogenic activity in animals was judged. Rinkus & Legator (1979) reviewed data from bacterial tests on 465 known or suspected carcinogens. The compounds were divided into a number of separate categories, depending on their chemical structure. The chemicals that showed the best correlation (94%) between mutagenic and carcinogenic activity were those that either could react directly with DNA (i.e., ultimate electrophiles) or could be activated by metabolic enzymes to DNA reactants. Chemicals that, from their structure, appeared unlikely to react with DNA, showed a very poor correlation between mutagenic and carcinogenic activity. These chemicals appear to cause cancer by a different, possibly non-genotoxic, mechanism.

The most ambitious validation exercise to date was the International Program for the Evaluation of Short-term Tests for Carcinogenicity (de Serres & Ashby, 1981) in which some thirty in vitro and in vivo assays involving more than fifty laboratories were evaluated for their ability to discriminate between carcinogenic and non-carcinogenic compounds. Twenty-five carcinogens and 17 non-carcinogens, including 14 pairs of carcinogenic/non-carcinogenic analogues, were tested in most of the assays. Animal cancer bioassay data from the 42 chemicals were critically evaluated by an expert committee. Bacterial mutation assays gave the best overall performance producing reliable results in a large number of laboratories, and were confirmed as the first choice as an initial screening test. However, it was also noted that some known rodent carcinogens were not detected or were only detected with difficulty by the standard Ames procedure. Other assays that discriminated well between carcinogens and non-carcinogens included in vitro tests for chromosome damage and unscheduled DNA synthesis and assays using yeasts, and, although the data-base was smaller, results from Drosophila tests and in vitro gene mutation assays suggested that they were useful components of a testing battery. In vivo tests for chromosome damage showed their ability to differentiate between a number of carcinogen/non-carcinogen pairs and thus confirmed their value for investigating the in vivo behaviour of chemicals found to be mutagenic in in vitro tests.

A further major collaborative study, which was designed to complement the International Program referred to above, was conducted under the auspices of the International Programme on Chemical Safety. The object of this project was to identify the best in vitro test or tests to complement the bacterial reversion assay (Ashby et al., 1985).

Although bacterial mutation assays have a high predictive value for carcinogenicity, in most validation studies at least 10% of compounds give results that conflict with the animal cancer data. For this reason, it is generally accepted that bacterial assays should not be used in isolation for the testing of chemicals and it is common practice to use a "battery" or "package" of short-term assays as a preliminary screen.

Carcinogenic and/or mutagenic chemicals may induce one or more of a number of genetic changes and an assessment of the possible genotoxic hazard posed by a chemical should normally contain assays capable of detecting changes at both the gene and chromosomal level, and in some cases, tests for DNA damage. Some authorities such as the Organisation for Economic Cooperation and Development (OECD), the European Economic Community (EEC) and the US Environmental Protection Agency (US EPA), require specific tests to be carried out on certain types of chemicals. The application and interpretation of short-term tests are discussed in detail in section 4 and additional information is presented by Dean et al. (1983).

Section 2 contains descriptions in phylogenetic order of the most commonly used and most widely-accepted assays, some of which, however, are used more often than others. In each procedure, specific minimal scientific and technical criteria can be identified that are critical factors in obtaining data of acceptable quality and reliability. These factors are emphasized in section 2 and should be carefully considered by scientists contemplating setting up a testing facility and by those who are responsible for judging the validity of submitted data and assessing the genotoxic hazard associated with the use of chemicals. Additional criteria that relate to good laboratory practice in genetic toxicology and to the type and quality of laboratory facilities are discussed in section 3.

2. DESCRIPTION OF WIDELY-ADOPTED PROCEDURES

2.1 Bacterial Mutation Assays

2.1.1 Principles and scientific basis of the assay

Bacteria have proved to be most suitable for the study of mutations, which are rare events, occurring naturally at a specific locus in less than one in a million bacteria at each cell division. However, as bacteria are single-celled organisms that divide rapidly and can be grown in large numbers in a few hours, it has proved to be relatively easy to grow tens of millions of organisms under circumstances where the one in a million event can be detected. Furthermore, a great deal is known about the biochemistry and genetics of bacteria, and it has, therefore, been possible to develop special strains that are sensitive to a wide range of mutagens.

Bacterial test systems fall into 3 main classes, namely, those that detect backward mutations, those that detect forward mutations, and those that rely on a DNA repair deficiency. By far the most widely-exploited method is the induction of backward or reverse mutations in Salmonella typhimurium or, less frequently, Escherichia coli. The important point of this type of test is that, from the very beginning, each strain of bacterium already possesses a selected mutation that prevents it performing an essential biochemical function, such as the synthesis of one out of the twenty or so amino acids necessary for the synthesis of proteins, unlike a non-mutant, "wild-type", strain of the same species. A wild-type (prototrophic) strain can synthesize all its amino acids from inorganic nitrogen (e.g., ammonium phosphate) when provided with a suitable source of carbon (e.g., glucose). The strains of S. typhimurium used in reverse mutation tests cannot synthesize the amino acid histidine and are therefore designated as "his⁻". Similarly, E. coli strains that cannot synthesize the amino acid tryptophan have been used and are referred to as "trp⁻". Such strains are said to be auxotrophic. The reverse mutation test is so named because it can show whether a test material can reverse the effect of the pre-existing mutation (e.g., his⁻) by causing a second mutation which allows the bacterium to synthesize histidine from inorganic nitrogen. This process is often abbreviated to "his⁻" to "his⁺" and is referred to a reversion from auxotrophy to prototrophy. The resulting mutants are also called revertants.

In order to make the test more sensitive, the tester strains have been made more susceptible to mutagens by genetically changing the structure of their cell walls so that

they become more permeable to large fat-soluble molecules.
Other genetic manipulations have reduced their ability to
repair regions of DNA that have been damaged by chemicals and
various types of radiation. Further sensitivity in the tester
strains has been attained by introducing plasmids (small DNA
molecules) that carry genes that interfere further with DNA
repair, making the host bacteria even more vulnerable to the
mutagenic effects of chemicals.

Because there are many different types of DNA damage, and
because the use of the reverse mutation test requires the test
chemical to hit a very small target in order to overcome the
effect of the pre-existing mutation, several different targets
are presented to the test chemical. This is achieved by using
several strains of the same species of bacterium, each one
carrying a different pre-existing mutation in the same
amino-acid gene. Two types of mutation are employed:
base-pair substitution and frameshift. For example, there are
several different mutations in the histidine gene of S.
typhimurium, each different mutation being carried in a
different strain, but all strains sharing the other traits
(e.g., DNA-repair defects and cell-wall defects that make them
very sensitive).

As mentioned in section 1, E. coli and S. typhimurium lack
most of the enzymes that can perform the type of metabolic
activation characteristic of mammalian biotransformation. The
enzymes are therefore added in the form of a liver extract
prepared from laboratory animals, usually rats. The rats are
given chemicals that increase the amount of
metabolic-activation enzymes in the liver and are then left
for a few days before they are killed, to allow the enzymes to
build up. This is known as induction, and the chemicals that
are used are called "inducers". The most widely used inducer
is Aroclor® 1254, a mixture of polychlorinated biphenyls.
Phenobarbital plus 5,6-benzoflavone is also used for
induction. The liver is ground up and centrifuged at high
speed; the supernatant liquid contains the metabolic enzymes
(some of which are bound to membranes (microsomes)) and is
called S9 (short for "9000 g supernatant").

In a bacterial mutation assay, his⁻ bacteria are mixed
with S9 and several doses of the test chemical and are allowed
to divide by providing a small amount of histidine. If the
test chemical is itself mutagenic, or if the enzymes in the S9
act on the test chemical to produce substances (metabolites)
that are mutagenic, this will be shown by the appearance of a
small proportion of bacteria, which will continue to grow and
divide, even when the supply of histidine has been used up.
These revertants can be detected easily, since their DNA has
been permanently changed so that they can make histidine from
inorganic nitrogen, and can grow indefinitely without added

histidine. Thus, each mutant eventually grows into a microscopic colony and it is the count of these that is the end-point of the assay.

2.1.2   Relevance and limitations of the assay

Bacterial mutation assays are used in a large number of laboratories throughout the world. Several large-scale trials, carried out to test the usefulness of these assays in detecting potential carcinogens and mutagens (Purchase et al., 1978; McMahon et al., 1979; Bartsch et al., 1980; de Serres & Ashby, 1981), have shown that bacterial mutation assays are very good at picking out chemicals known to cause cancer. Moreover, relatively few chemicals that do not cause cancer have given positive results in these tests. In general, therefore, chemicals that are mutagenic in bacteria are more likely to cause cancer than chemicals that are not mutagenic, i.e., mutagenicity is a characteristic property of a large number of carcinogens. It is important to understand, however, that there does not seem to be any useful quantitative relationship between the ability of a chemical to cause mutations in bacteria and cancer in animals or people. In other words, a chemical that is a strong mutagen in bacteria is not necessarily a strong carcinogen in animals, nor is it always the case that a weak bacterial mutagen will be a weak carcinogen.

A second limitation of bacterial mutation tests is their inability to detect chemicals that are thought to induce cancer, not by causing DNA damage, but by other means, as yet poorly understood. Such substances include asbestos, nickel, arsenic, and hormone-like chemicals such as diethylstilboestrol. There are other substances, e.g., phorbol esters, which are extracts of certain species of the plant genus Euphorbia, and certain secondary bile acids, which usually do not cause cancer when given alone to animals, but which increase the effects of other cancer-causing chemicals. This so-called tumour promotion does not come about because of the production of DNA damage. Thus, it will not be detected by mutagenicity assays which detect only substances that can initiate cancer. Nevertheless, promoters may well play a significant part in human cancer and it is important to recognise that bacterial mutagenicity tests cannot detect promoting activity.

Substances are known that cause genetic defects (and possibly cancer) in higher organisms by interfering with the machinery that controls the exact distribution of chromosome sets from one generation of cells to the next, and from parents to children, causing mistakes in the number and structure of chromosomes delivered to cells during cell

division. Such substances do not always cause DNA damage, and
will not be detected in bacterial mutagenicity tests, since
bacteria do not have chromosomes.

The use of cell-free extracts (S9) from rats to represent
the metabolism of chemicals in mammals is another limitation
that must be borne in mind, when interpreting the results of
bacterial mutation tests. Studies have shown that breaking up
liver cells can, in some cases, distort the pattern of
metabolism, resulting in levels and proportions of metabolites
that would not be produced in the intact liver. Moreover,
because the test is carried out in a test-tube rather than in
an animal, it is impossible to allow for several other
factors, which can in some cases give a misleading impression
of the mutagenic or carcinogenic effects of a chemical. The
way the chemical enters the body and is distributed to the
various organs, how each organ metabolises it, and how the
chemical or its metabolites leave the body can all play a part
in determining if, and to what extent, the chemical is
mutagenic or carcinogenic for the animal. None of these
factors can be reproduced in a test-tube containing bacteria,
S9, and a chemical.

Despite these limitations, bacterial mutation tests have
been found by trial and error to be extremely valuable as the
first in a series of tests for screening chemicals for
potential mutagenic and carcinogenic activity. Moreover,
bacterial tests have been validated in far greater detail than
any other tests currently used in genetic toxicology.

2.1.3   The procedure

The bacterial mutation test that forms the basis of all
screening programmes was devised by B.N. Ames and his
co-workers and is usually referred to as the
"Salmonella/microsome test". It is essential that workers who
intend to use this test, and those who review the results of
such tests read the following papers: Ames et al. (1975),
McCann et al. (1975), McCann & Ames (1976), Maron et al.
(1981), Levin et al. (1982), and Maron & Ames (1984). The
following technical details are not intended as a defined
recommended protocol, but represent good current practice and
good criteria for successful bacterial tests.

2.1.3.1   Outline of the basic procedure

In the Salmonella/microsome test, several his⁻ strains
of S. typhimurium are used in order to detect several
different types of DNA damage. A set of sterile test-tubes is
held at 45 °C. Molten soft agar ("top agar") (2 ml)
containing a low concentration of histidine is added to each

tube followed by 0.1 ml of a culture of the required bacterial strain, which has been grown over the previous night in a very rich nutrient liquid ("nutrient broth"). This "overnight culture" contains about 1×10^9 bacteria per ml, so that each tube contains about 1×10^8 bacteria. A range of doses of the test chemical (dissolved in a suitable solvent) is then added, each dose to a separate tube. Dimethylsulfoxide (DMSO) is the most widely used solvent. It dissolves numerous different kinds of chemicals, is miscible with water and, at the amount used in the test (0.1 ml or less), is not toxic to bacteria.

Several tubes are set aside to act as "controls", i.e., tubes that will receive the solvent but not the test chemical and will therefore indicate the background (spontaneous) level of mutation. It is essential to know the level of background mutation for each bacterial strain in each experiment in order to tell whether the test chemical has had any mutagenic effect. Finally, 0.5 ml of S9-mix is added to each tube and the contents mixed thoroughly by rapid shaking. S9-mix consists of S9 (usually between 4 and 30% by volume) to which has been added nicotinamide-adenine dinucleotide phosphate (NADP) and glucose-6-phosphate (which together provide energy for metabolism), phosphate buffer to maintain pH, and salts of magnesium and potassium. A set of tubes is also prepared without S9. This is to check whether the test chemical can cause mutation without the need for metabolic activation. Chemicals of this type are directly-acting mutagens: certain directly-acting mutagens can be made non-mutagenic by S9; thus, it is important to include this check.

The additions of bacteria, test chemical, and S9-mix are made in rapid succession, in order to avoid the potentially harmful effects of the rather high temperature (45 °C) necessary to keep the soft agar molten. As soon as possible after mixing, the contents of each tube are poured on to the surface of 30 ml of solid 1.5% agar ("bottom agar") which contains glucose, ammonium and other salts, and phosphate buffer in a 9-cm petri dish ("plate"). The plate is shaken to distribute the top agar in a thin, even layer over the bottom agar. The lid of the plate is replaced and each plate is placed on a level surface: the top agar then cools and solidifies. When all the tubes have been poured, and the plates have cooled, they are inverted and placed in an incubator at 37 °C for 48 h.

This is called the plate incorporation technique, since all the ingredients of the test are incorporated into a thin layer of soft agar on the surface of harder agar in a plate. During the first few hours of incubation, all the his⁻ bacteria will grow, since there is a trace of histidine present. At the same time that the bacteria are dividing, the enzymes in the S9-mix, supported by the energy provided by the NADP and G-6-P, may act on the test chemical to form metabolites that can enter the rapidly dividing bacteria. Some of these metabolites, or the test chemical itself, may react with the bacterial DNA, causing DNA damage, some of which will lead to mutation in a very small fraction of the progeny of the 100 million bacteria present at the start of incubation. When all the histidine has been used up, the bulk of bacteria will stop dividing, and a thin, visible confluent lawn of bacteria will have formed in the soft agar. However, bacteria that have sustained DNA damage leading to a mutation with the effect of reverting the his⁻ gene to his⁺ will continue to divide, since they can now synthesize their own histidine from the ammonium salts in the bottom agar. Each single revertant his⁺ (mutant) bacterium can produce enough daughter bacteria in 48 h to form a single colony of bacteria, easily visible to the naked eye. Therefore, the number of such colonies on the plate is an accurate reflection of the number of his⁺ revertants that have arisen spontaneously or by the action of the test chemical. If there are significantly more revertant colonies on treated plates than on control (solvent only) plates, and if the numbers of revertants rise with increasing dose, the result of the test is positive, and the chemical is a bacterial mutagen.

2.1.3.2 Critical factors in the procedure

There are several conditions that must be met in order to ensure an adequate test: these are briefly discussed below. More extensive discussion can be found in IARC (1980a) and Venitt et al. (1983).

Base-line protocol

It is essential that a base-line protocol should be written before starting a screening programme. Methods for the preparation and storage of S9 and bacterial strains, and other procedures should be thoroughly checked by performing assays with reference mutagens and authenticated bacterial strains, under conditions prescribed by the chosen protocol. Advice should be sought from experienced investigators.

Choice, checking, storage, and culture of bacterial strains

The following strains of S. typhimurium are most-commonly used for routine screening (Ames et al., 1975): TA 1535, TA 1538, TA 98, and TA 100. Strains TA 97 and TA 102 are also considered useful, under some circumstances (Maron & Ames, 1983). In addition, E. coli WP2uvrApKM101 is often included.

This trp⁻ strain is very sensitive to a wide range of mutagens (McMahon et al., 1979; de Serres & Ashby, 1981; Matsushima et al., 1981; Venitt & Crofton-Sleigh, 1981).

Bacterial strains should be regularly checked for their characteristic genetic traits, including: amino acid requirement; background mutation; induced mutation with reference mutagens; presence of plasmids where appropriate; presence of cell-wall and DNA-repair mutations.

Authenticated "master cultures" should be stored at a temperature below -70 °C. Overnight cultures for routine assays should be prepared by inoculation from master cultures or from plates made from a master culture - never from a previously-used overnight culture. The overnight culture should contain at least 10^9 viable bacteria per ml, and should be freshly prepared for each experiment.

Negative and positive controls

Each assay should include negative controls (addition of the solvent but no test chemical) in order to check the background mutation and positive controls (addition of reference mutagens to check that the assay is performing correctly). A list of appropriate positive control mutagens is given by Maron & Ames (1984). Where possible, the compounds selected as positive controls should be structurally related to the compound under test.

Test material and solvents

All data available on the substance to be tested should be provided and recorded, including its lot or batch number, physical appearance, chemical structure, purity, solubility, reactivity in aqueous and non-aqueous solvents, temperature- and pH-stability, and sensitivity to light. A sample of each substance to be assayed for mutagenicity should be retained for reference purposes.

Solutions of test substances should be freshly prepared for each experiment, and unused portions should be discarded. The nature and percentage of impurities should be given: if a known impurity is present in the test substance, it too should be assayed for mutagenicity at doses equivalent to those that would be present in the chosen doses of the major constituent. If a mixture is to be tested, this should be stated.

The proposed uses of the test substance should be known, since antibiotics, surfactants, preservatives, and biocides pose special problems in bacterial mutation assays.

It is essential to devise operating procedures that minimize the hazards from storage, handling, weighing, pipetting, and disposing of mutagens and carcinogens, and that deal with accidental contamination (Montesano et al., 1979; IARC, 1980b; University of Birmingham, 1980; MRC, 1981). Laboratories should follow the guidelines laid down for Good Laboratory Practice (GLP) (PMAA, 1976; Federal Register, 1978). These important matters are discussed further in section 3.

In most cases, DMSO is the best solvent, but, in cases where it is unsuitable, other solvents may be used (Maron et al., 1981).

Preparation and use of S9

The animals should be free of disease and infection, kept clean and at a reasonable temperature and should not be stressed by careless handling. Dosing with inducing agents should be consistent from one batch of animals to the next. Animals should be killed humanely and the livers removed and chilled as soon as possible. S9 should be stored at, or below, -70 °C.

Optimum mutagenesis with a particular test compound depends on the amount of S9 added per plate. Too much as well as too little S9 can drastically lower the sensitivity of the test. The optimum S9 level for a given compound should therefore be checked. The amount of S9 per plate is best expressed as mg liver protein per plate calculated from the protein concentration of the S9.

There are two widely-accepted methods of using S9-mix:

(a) S9-mix is mixed with the top agar, bacteria, and test substance, and the whole mixture is immediately poured on to the surface of the bottom agar (Ames et al., 1975); and

(b) in the pre-incubation method, the test substance, bacteria, and S9-mix are mixed and incubated for 30 min; top agar is then added, and the mixture is poured on to the bottom agar. This modification is often more efficient in detecting certain classes of mutagens, for example, aliphatic N-nitroso compounds (Bartsch et al., 1976; Yahagi et al., 1977).

Design of experiments

A minimum of three plates per dose should be used in all experiments. Doses of test chemicals should be spaced at intervals differing by factors of less than 5. Narrow spacing of doses avoids missing mutagens that are very toxic and that produce very steep dose-response curves with sharp cut-offs. Combining the requirement for narrow spacing of doses with the need to encompass a very wide range of doses, two strategies emerge:

(a)   a large experiment with closely-spaced doses ranging from sub-microgram to milligram levels, using 7 or 8 doses together with positive and solvent controls; and

(b)   two experiments, the first using submicrogram to tens or hundreds of micrograms. If the results are positive, this should be confirmed in the strains and the dose range in which the positive effect was observed. If negative results are obtained, the second experiment should be carried out at a higher dose range, using the highest dose from the first experiment as the lowest dose in the second experiment, and extending the dose-range well into the milligram range.

All experiments should be repeated at least once. If the first experiment produces a weak or equivocal result (e.g., a dose-related but less than 2-fold increase in revertants per plate), the experiment should be repeated until a consistent picture emerges.

Incubation and examination of plates

Plates should be incubated at 37 °C for at least 48 h before being scored. It is important to ensure that volatile test compounds and gases are incubated in closed systems. After incubation, it is essential to inspect the background lawn of both treated and control plates with a dissecting microscope in order to check for toxic effects (thinning of the lawn) or excess growth, which may indicate the presence of amino acids in the test material.

2.1.4   Presentation and interpretation of data

2.1.4.1 Data-processing and presentation

The description of the protocol should be detailed enough to allow independent replication of the assay. If a published protocol has been used, this should be referred to, and any deviations from it should be indicated. The following information should be included in reports: source of the S9 (strain and species of animal); details of inducers; percentage of S9 in the S9-mix; mg liver protein per plate; concentration of buffer and cofactors; items bought in from proprietary sources (e.g., S9, ready-poured plates) should be noted. "Raw" data should be provided: individual values of numbers of mutant colonies per plate should be tabulated in ascending order of dose, starting with the solvent controls. Data from positive controls should be clearly identified and separated from the results obtained for the test substance. The doses of test compound should be expressed by weight per plate and not by volume. If the test substance is a formulation or mixture, results should also be expressed per weight of active ingredient(s). Providing that a complete raw data set is provided, it is also useful to present graphs showing dose-response curves.

2.1.4.2 Interpretation of data in terms of positive and negative

For a substance to be considered positive in a plate-incorporation test it should have induced a dose-related and statistically significant increase in mutations compared with appropriate concurrent controls, in one or more strains of bacteria, in the presence and/or absence of S9, in at least two separate experiments. Experience has shown that a doubling or more of the background mutation, combined with a dose-response curve, indicates a positive response.

A test substance is considered negative if it does not produce any increase in mutation at any dose, in at least 2 separate experiments that complied with the base-line protocol submitted with the test report. This protocol should include the following requirements: the strains used, e.g., S. typhimurium strains TA 1535, TA 1538, TA 98, TA 100; E. coli uvrA(pKM101)); testing at doses spaced at 4-fold intervals or less and extending to the limits imposed by toxicity or solubility, or, where the substance is very soluble, into the milligram range; adequate concurrent negative and positive controls, including positive controls to test the efficiency of the S9-mix; tests in the presence and absence of S9-mix; and finally, evidence of the identity of the bacterial strains used in each experiment.

2.1.4.3 Dealing with ambiguous results

An ambiguous result arises when, at one or more doses, there are more revertants per plate than are seen on concurrent control plates, but there is not a clear dose-response relationship. This increase may be consistent in two or more experiments. The effect might occur in just one tester strain and at one particular level of S9 in the S9-mix. Such a result cannot be classified as negative, neither is it positive. The use of historical control values to interpret ambiguous results is not recommended.

Ambiguous results may be caused by a technical problem, such as the presence of nutrients in the test substance or the bacteriostatic effect of the test substance; or it might be an indication that a change in experimental procedure is required. In addition, in the course of several replicate experiments, one or two assays might be positive, and some might be negative. Results of this type may be classified as "irreproducible". Under these circumstances, the use of alternative protocols may resolve the problem. See Venitt et al. (1983) for further discussion.

2.1.5 Discussion

2.1.5.1 How the most critical factors identified above can influence the validity of the data

The conduct of bacterial mutation tests requires close attention to every aspect of the experimental procedure. Success in running large numbers of such tests in routine screening programmes depends on the establishment of consistent methods for every phase of the experiment. A deficiency in just one area will jeopardize the whole enterprise.

2.1.5.2 Interpretation of the results in terms of the intrinsic mutagenic activity of the test material

A bacterial mutagenicity assay simply determines whether the substance under investigation is or is not a bacterial mutagen in the presence and/or absence of an exogenous metabolizing system derived from a mammal (S9). Such a test cannot determine whether the test substance is mutagenic and/or carcinogenic in any other species. However, it may be concluded that a substance found to be mutagenic in properly-conducted bacterial mutation assays should be regarded as potentially mutagenic or carcinogenic for mammals (including man) until further evidence indicates otherwise.

2.2 Genotoxicity Studies Using Yeast Cultures

2.2.1 Introduction

The budding and fission yeasts Saccharomyces cerevisiae and Schizosaccharomyces pombe, respectively, are among the most extensively studied of the eukaryotes and provide convenient tools for use in genetic toxicology studies of environmental chemicals. The internal structure of the yeast cells shows strong similarities to that of the cells of higher organisms, in that they possess a differentiated nucleus containing a nucleolus. The accurate functioning of cell division depends on the synthesis of a spindle apparatus; however, unlike mammalian cells, yeasts and other fungi maintain their nuclear membrane during cell division.

The budding and fission yeasts are distantly related and differ significantly in the persistance of the diploid phase of the life cycle. S. cerevisiae haploid strains of the a and mating type, and diploid cultures heterozygous and homozygous for mating-type may be cultivated in the vegetative phase. In contrast, in S. pombe, the vegetative haploid cells of mating type h^+ and h^- fuse to produce a zygote, which undergoes immediate reduction division (meiosis) to produce 4-spored haploid asci. Thus, S. cerevisiae strains are suitable for routine use as both vegetative haploids and diploids, whereas S. pombe strains are suitable for use only for the measurement of genetic end-points detectable in haploids. Diploid vegetative cultures of S. pombe have been produced by special treatments but have not been used in genotoxicity studies so far.

Yeasts are physiologically-robust organisms, tolerating pH values between 3 and 9; they survive at temperatures from freezing to above 40 °C, and growth can occur over a range of approximately 18 °C - 40 °C. Growth is optimal at 28 °C and 32 °C for S. cerevisiae and S. pombe, respectively, using a carbon source such as glucose.

Diploid cultures of S. cerevisiae undergo meiosis under a variety of conditions, such as those found in exhausted medium and in the presence of 1% potassium acetate. Thus, by varying the medium, it is possible to study S. cerevisiae during both mitotic and meiotic cell division. The uncontrolled induction of meiosis and spore formation in exhausted vegetative growth medium can lead to problems during long periods of treatment. Such problems are eliminated by the use of diploid strains such as JDI (described later), which are unable to undergo meiosis and spore formation.

For both fission and budding yeast, there is an extensive data-base of experiments involving their use in studies on the genotoxicity of chemicals. This data base has been reviewed by the US Environmental Protection Agency Gene-Tox Program (Loprieno et al., 1983; Zimmermann et al., 1984). However, readers should be aware that significant numbers of chemicals in the yeast data base were screened prior to the introduction of techniques involving in vitro mammalian activation mixes. Thus, many of the apparently negative results in the literature may stem from the use of unsuitable protocols.

The primary advantages of yeasts in genotoxicity studies can be summarized as follows:

    (a)   eukaryotic chromosome organization;
    (b)   variety of genetic end-points can be assayed;

(c) cost-effective assays requiring limited technical and laboratory facilities using a "robust" organism.

2.2.2 Genetic end-points

When used in genotoxicity studies, yeast cultures have significant advantages over other test systems in terms of the comprehensive range of genetic end-points that can be assayed. These end-points include:

(a) point mutation in chromosomal and mitochondrial genes;
(b) recombination, both between and within genes; and
(c) chromosome aneuploidy during both mitosis and meiosis.

A number of other variables including membrane damage, differential killing in repair-deficient strains, and selective effects have also been studied. However, the data base for such events is still limited, and this section will be confined to the events classified into groups (a), (b), and (c).

2.2.2.1 Point mutation

A variety of forward mutation systems has been used with yeast cultures. However, the most extensively studied system has been the one based on the induction of defective alleles of the genes for adenine synthesis. The system involves the use of cultures carrying defective mutations of the genes Adenine-1 and Adenine-2 of S. cerevisiae and Adenine-6 and Adenine-7 of S. pombe, the presence of which results in the production of red-pigmented colonies in S. cerevisiae and red/purple colonies in S. pombe, owing to the presence of an intracellular pigment (aminoimidazole carboxylic acid ribonucleotide in the case of adenine-2 mutations).

Forward mutations are detected in such strains by the induction of further mutations at 5 genes that precede the production of the red/purple pigment in the adenine synthetic pathway. Such mutations result in the production of doubly-defective colonies, which can be visually observed as white colonies or sectors. The system can be illustrated as shown below:

Strain P_1 of S. pombe genotype: ade6-60, rad10-198,h⁻

```
ade6-60          ----------------→   ade6-60 ade x  <- new mutation
red/purple       forward mutation       white
colonies         produced by both     colonies
                 base-substitution
                 and frameshift
                 mutagenesis
```

The assay involves the treatment of red/purple cultures with the test agent and the visual screening of colonies produced on low-adenine medium for the production of whole white or sectored colonies (Loprieno, 1981).

The most widely-used yeast strain for the detection of reverse mutation is the haploid strain of S. cerevisiae XV185-14C, developed by von Borstel and his colleagues (Mehta & von Borstel, 1981), which has the following genotype:

a ade2-1, arg4-17, lys1-1, trp5-48, his1-7, hom3-10

The markers ade2-1, arg4-17, lys1-1, try5-48 are ochre "nonsense" mutations, which are revertible by base-substitution mutagens that induce site-specific mutations or ochre-suppressor mutations in t-RNA loci. The marker his1-7 is a missense mutation that is reverted mainly by second site mutations; hom3-10 is believed to be a frameshift defect because of its response to a range of diagnostic mutagens. As with most, if not all, of the frameshift mutations identified in yeast, the hom3-10 allele reverts at a relatively low frequency and its use in testing protocols requires the screening of large populations of cells.

In diploid strains of S. cerevisiae, the only mutation marker that has been extensively used is the ilv1-92 mutation that is present in the homoallelic condition in strain D7. Unfortunately, the marker responds to only a limited range of mutagens and it would be inappropriate to regard it as a comprehensive point mutation screening system for environmental chemicals.

The induction of mutations that lead to defects in mitochondrial function in yeast may be detected by the assay of the frequency of respiration-deficient "petite" colonies, which are incapable of aerobic respiration. Such colonies are characterized by their small size and their inability to grow on non-fermentable carbon sources such as glycerol. Petite colonies may be produced by the induction of both chromosomal and extrachromosomal events but, in diploid cells, those detected are predominantly of extrachromosomal origin. In yeasts, extrachromosomal mutations are induced at high levels by a wide range of chemical mutagens. However, at present, the significance of such events is far from clear (Wilkie & Gooneskera, 1980).

2.2.2.2 Recombination[a]

In eukaryotic cells, genetic exchanges between homologous chromosomes are generally confined to a specialized stage of meiotic cell division which, in yeasts, occurs during the process of sporulation. Recombinational events in yeasts may also be detected during mitotic or vegetative division, though the spontaneous frequency is generally at least 1000 times less than that observed during meiosis. Sporulating yeast cultures can be used to study the rates of both spontaneous and induced meiotic recombination, but it is generally the mitotic events that are of practical value in genotoxicity studies.

Mitotic recombination can be detected in yeasts both between genes and within genes. The former event is called mitotic crossing-over and generates reciprocal products whereas the latter is most frequently non-reciprocal and is called gene conversion. Crossing-over is generally assayed by the production of recessive homozygous colonies or sectors produced in a heterogenous strain. Gene conversion is assayed by the production of prototrophic revertants produced in a heteroallelic strain carrying two different defective alleles of the same gene. Mitotic gene conversion can be distinguished functionally from point mutation by the elevated levels of prototrophy produced in heteroallelic strains compared with levels in homoallelic strains (carrying two copies of the same mutation).

The value of assaying mitotic recombination in yeast in genotoxicity studies stems from the observation that both

----

[a] Nomenclature

Genetic loci in this paper are labelled as follows:

abbreviation for gene

ade 6 - 60

specific   mutant
gene   number

Capital letters indicate the wild-type form of the gene and lower case the mutant form. The suffixes r and s indicate resistance and sensitivity to antimicrobial agents, respectively.

rad loci - indicate genes involved in DNA repair.

●——— represents a chromosome with its centromere.

events are elevated by exposure to genotoxic chemicals. These increases are produced in a non-specific manner, i.e., levels are increased by all types of mutagens, irrespective of their mode of action. Thus, the primary advantage of assaying for the induction of mitotic recombination is that the events involved are reflective of the cell's response to a wide spectrum of genetic damage. A number of suitable strains of S. cerevisiae have been constructed for use in genotoxicity testing. However, for the purposes of this document it will be confined to those most frequently used and convenient for use.

Mitotic gene conversion can be assayed using selective medium in the diploid S. cerevisiae strain D4 (Zimmermann, 1975). The genotype of D4 is as follows:

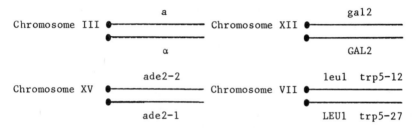

ade2-2, ade2-1, trp5-12, and trp5-27 are heteroalleles at the ADE2 and TRP5 loci, respectively. These alleles undergo mitotic gene conversion to produce prototrophic colonies carrying one wild-type allele which makes growth possible on selective medium lacking either tryptophan or adenine, e.g.,

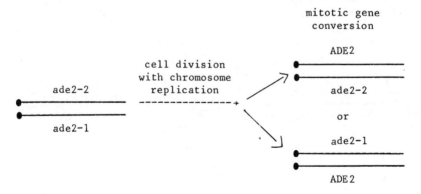

The D4 strain has been extensively used in the study of genotoxic chemicals (Zimmermann et al., 1984) and has proved to be a valuable tool. However, the use of the strain is

limited by the relatively high spontaneous reversion frequencies of the ADE-2 marker which means that, if this loci is to be used, cultures with low spontaneous prototroph frequency must be selected prior to chemical treatment.

Mitotic gene conversion can also be assayed in the strain JDI (Sharp & Parry, 1981), which is capable of simultaneously assaying mitotic crossing-over on chromosome XV. The genotype of JDI is as follows:

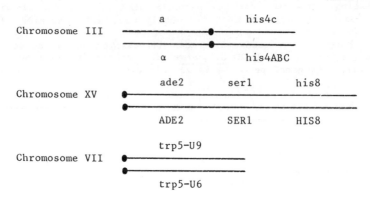

his4C, his4ABC, trp-U9, and trp5-U6 are heteroalleles at the HIS4 and TRP5 loci, respectively. These alleles undergo mitotic gene conversion to produce proto colonies carrying one wild-type allele which makes growth possible on selective medium lacking either tryptophan or histidine. Mitotic crossing-over can be assayed by the production of red colonies or sectors homozygous for ade-2 and the markers distal on chromosome XV, e.g.,

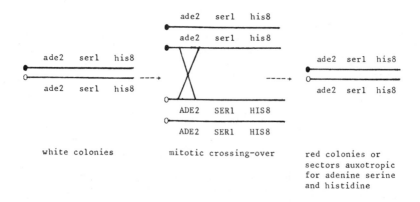

Thus, using the strain <u>JDI</u>, it is possible to assay mitotic gene conversion at two separate loci and also to detect one of the possible homozygous chromosome combinations produced by mitotic crossing-over (but not both reciprocal products). The strain has been selected for its inability to undergo sporulation and is thus suitable for long periods of treatment. Protocols are available for the use of this strain under conditions of optimal cytochrome P-450 concentrations (Kelly & Parry, 1983a).

A particularly convenient multipurpose strain of <u>S. cerevisiae</u> is D7 (Zimmermann, 1975) which carries a set of genetic markers that allow the simultaneous assay of mitotic crossing-over, gene conversion, and point mutation.

The genotype of D7 is as follows:

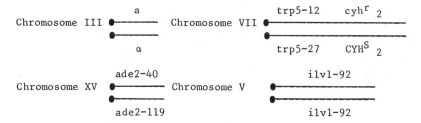

The heteroalleles of the <u>TRP-5</u> locus, <u>tryp5-12</u> and <u>trp5-27</u>, undergo mitotic gene conversion to produce proto-trophic colonies carrying one wild-type allele which makes growth possible on selective medium lacking tryptophan. While <u>ade2-40</u> is a completely inactive allele of <u>ADE-2</u> that produces deep red colonies, <u>ade2-119</u> is a leaky allele (only partially defective) causing accumulation of only a small amount of pigment and thus producing pink colonies. In heteroallelic diploids, the <u>ade2-40</u> and <u>ade-2-119</u> alleles complement to give rise to white adenine-independent colonies. Mitotic crossing-over in <u>D7</u> may give rise to the production of cells homoallelic for the <u>ade2</u> mutations and thus lead to the observation of both red and pink reciprocal products, e.g.,

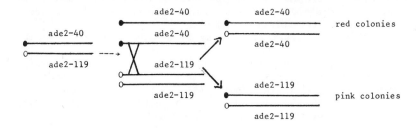

The frequency of induced reciprocal mitotic crossing-over can be unambiguously confirmed in D7 by the visual observation of treated colonies. Mitotic crossing-over can also be assayed in D7 by the use of the recessive cycloheximide resistant cyh^r_2 allele on chromosome VII. Crossing over between CYH_2 and the centromere of chromosome VII results in the production of colonies that are capable of growth on medium containing cycloheximide (Kunz et al., 1980), e.g.,

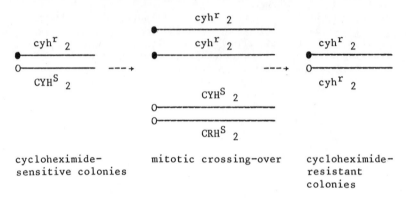

cycloheximide-   mitotic crossing-over   cycloheximide-
sensitive colonies   resistant
                                                       colonies

The final genetic event that can be asayed in strain D7 is the induction of base-substitution mutation at the homallelic -ilv1-92 markers by the production of prototrophs that grow on selective minimal media that lack isoleucine.

2.2.2.3 Aneuploidy

Abnormal chromosome segregations leading to the production of numerical chromosome aberrations can be detected in yeasts by genetic means using appropriate yeast strains. Suitable strains of S. cerevisiae are available that are capable of detecting and quantifying the reduction of monosomy (chromosome loss) during mitotic cell division from the 2n to the 2n-1 condition and the production of disomy (chromosome gain) and diploidisation in spores produced during meiotic cell division (sporulation) (Fig. 1).

Although a number of strains have been developed for the detection by genetic means of chromosome aneuploidy, only two have been extensively used in the screening of environmental chemicals. These are D_6 described by Parry & Zimmermann (1976) and DIS13 described by Sora et al. (1982), which have been developed for the assay of induced aneuploidy during mitotic and meiotic cell division, respectively.

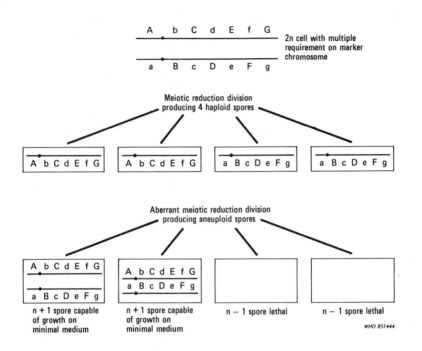

Fig. 1. Production of aneuploid spores in meiotic reduction division in the yeast Saccharomyces cerevisiae.

The genotype of S. cerevisiae diploid strain D6 is as follows:

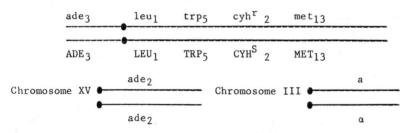

This strain forms red colonies because of the presence of ade₂ in a homozygous condition and is sensitive to the presence of cycloheximide in the medium because the cyh^r_2 resistance allele is recessive. The loss of the chromosome VII homologue carrying the dominant wild-type allele of this group of linked markers results in cells that form white (due to the expression of ade3) and cycloheximide-resistant (due to the expression of the selective cyh^r_2 marker) colonies that also express the markers leu_1, trp_5 and met_{13} (defined as G_o). Treatment protocols may involve the treatment of stationary phase cells in an appropriate buffer, exponential phase cells in buffer for a short period before they enter G_o, or growing cells in nutrient medium or on overlay plates.

The vast majority of the experimental studies on chemical mutagens using yeasts have involved liquid-suspension assays. Plate assays are nevertheless also possible and have been used for the assay of mitotic crossing-over, point mutation, and gene conversion (Fink & Lowenstein, 1971; Parry et al., 1976; Kunz et al., 1980). The advantages of liquid-suspension assays with regard to their ability to quantify cellular toxicity has, however, led to a preponderance of the studies in the literature. Cells of both yeast species have also been used extensively in host-mediated assays (Fahrig 1975; Loprieno et al., 1976) where they appear to tolerate incubation in mammals for long periods without eliciting host reactions.

Liquid-suspension assays involve treatment of cells with test chemicals for periods of preferably less than 24 h, removal of the test chemical, followed by plating on nutrient and selective medium for quantitation of both cell viability and the genetic end-point. Appropriate treatment media for the strains described here can be found in the publications of Loprieno, (1981), Mehta & von Borstel (1981), Parry & Sharp (1981), Sharp & Parry (1981), and Zimmermann & Scheel (1981) for both S. pombe and S. cerevisiae. Specific stages of mitotic cell division such as G_1, S, and G_2, can be investigated using synchronized cultures or, more conveniently, the separation of exponential phase cells by means of a zonal rotor (Davies et al., 1978).

Exposure of yeast cells to test chemicals is generally performed at the optimal growth temperature for the two species, i.e., 28 °C and 30 °C for S. cerevisiae and S. pombe, respectively. When mammalian metabolic activation preparations are used (see later) it may be appropriate to incubate cultures at 37 °C for a proportion of the total treatment time. In all such treatments, it is essential that media are adequately buffered at pH 7.0, as yeast cultures rapidly acidify their media. However, advantage can be taken of the pH tolerance of the organisms for the testing of chemicals that are biologically active at acid pHs. When

direct comparisons have been made between liquid yeast
suspension assays and bacterial plate assays, there has been a
close similarity in the sensitivity of the two assays (Parry &
Wilcox, 1982).

The assessment of the genotoxicity of chemicals in yeasts
during meiosis involves the treatment of cells during the
process of sporulation. Sporulation can be induced by the
transfer of vegetative cultures to a medium containing only
potassium acetate, but maximum levels of sporulation are
obtained if the culture is pre-grown in a pre-sporulation
medium containing both acetate and nutrients. Chemicals can
be assayed by exposure of cells throughout the sporulation
period or by treatment at specific stages during meiosis.
Suitable protocols for the assay of the effects of chemicals,
during meiosis, on mutation and chromosome aneuploidy have
been described in detail by Kelly & Parry (1983b) and Parry &
Parry (1983), respectively. During sporulation, the treatment
medium undergoes an alkaline pH change which may result in the
detoxification of some test compounds.

Mammalian metabolic activation preparations have been
employed in the assay of genotoxic chemicals using both
fission and budding yeasts, and suitable formulae for such
mixes have been described by Loprieno (1981) and Sharp & Parry
(1981), for use with Schizosaccharomyces amd Saccharomyces,
respectively. Most preparations are based on those used in
bacterial assays, which have been described earlier in this
report. Relatively few studies have been performed with
yeasts using various enzyme-inducing agents, mammalian
species, and liver fractions, though there is considerable
scope for such studies (Wilcox et al., 1982). There is now
evidence that, unlike Salmonella, yeast cells have a
significant endogenous metabolic capacity of their own (Callen
& Philpot, 1977) and protocols have been developed that
produce relatively high levels of cytochrome P-450 for periods
of up to 18 h of chemical treatment (Kelly & Parry, 1983a).

In yeast liquid-suspension assays, the time of exposure to
the test chemical depends on the nature of the protocols used,
the specific chemical being tested, and the yeast strain and
genetic end-point being studied. Thus, no specific
recommendations can be made with regard to the optimal time of
exposure required to adequately test chemicals. There are a
number of factors that should nevertheless be borne in mind
when designing an experiment:

(a) In studies with vegetative cells, care must be taken
     that, when diploid cells are used, the exposure times
     are not such as to lead to the induction of
     sporulation. If long exposure times are necessary,

cells should be checked for spore formation or use
made of non-sporulating strains such as JDI.

(b)   Exposure times should be sufficient to allow for
      entry of the test chemical into the cell and the
      production of the damage that provides the substrate
      for the induction of the specific end-point being
      assayed.

(c)   Provision must be made to allow for the expression of
      the end-point, e.g., in the case of the assay of
      induced chromosome aneuploidy a period of
      post-treatment cell division must take place before
      exposure to a selective agent.

Dose selection is another parameter that is highly
dependent on a number of experimental variables such as: the
culture used, the end-point measured and the nature of the
chemical being tested. In general, dose ranges should be
selected on the basis of cytotoxicity and solubility to
include concentrations that range from the "no-effect" dose
level up to 90% cell lethality with approximately 1/3 log
spacing. Dose selection is more difficult with assays such as
that for chromosome loss where "humped" dose-response curves
are a common feature (Parry et al., 1980) and maximum
induction of the end-point may occur at non-toxic doses.
Similar problems of dose selection have also been encountered
with specific chemicals such as the dinitropyrenes, whereas in
yeasts, the induction of mitotic gene conversion is detectable
only at non-toxic doses and is reduced at higher
concentrations (Wilcox & Parry, 1981). In such cases, there
is probably no alternative but to test a chemical down to
arbitrary concentrations of at least 0.1 μg/ml or to relate
the minimum test concentrations to potential exposure levels.
        After exposure to the test chemical, yeast cells are
washed and plated after dilution on nutrient medium and the
appropriate screening medium for the end-point under test. In
the case of cell viability and genetic end-points that provide
a large number of scorable events per plate, 3 replicate
plates are appropriate. However, in the case of relatively
rare events, such as mutation in frameshift marker strains,
and non-selectable events, such as forward mutation at the
adenine loci, the plate numbers must be increased to ensure
the statistical significance of the data, as with small
numbers the standard deviation of the plate counts will be
large. There is no generally agreed method of analysing the
data generated by yeast genotoxicity tests and a number of
suitable methods have been described, e.g., Loprieno et al.
(1976), Sharp & Parry, (1981), and Kelly & Parry (1983a).

It is essential that all experiments using yeast cells should be independently repeated and ambiguous results may require further experimentation with careful selection of sample size, treatment concentrations, culture stage, or metabolic activation system. The aims of such repeated experiments should be to increase the statistical validity of the results.

2.2.3 Information required

Data are best presented in tabular form supplemented with the appropriate graphical treatment. A test report should include the following information:

(a) strain of yeast used and genotype;

(b) description of the test conditions, including growth phase of cells used, whether growing or non-growing; details should be provided of length of treatment, dose levels, toxicity, medium, and treatment procedure; the negative and positive controls used should be clearly specified;

(c) raw data should be provided to include plate counts of viability and colony type selected, calculations of survival and frequency of genetic end-point under study, and dose-response relationships if applicable; and

(d) the results should be evaluated using an appropriate statistical procedure and interpretation provided.

2.2.4 Interpretation

2.2.4.1 Significance of positive results in yeast assays

1. A positive response in mutation assays is indicative of the ability of a chemical to induce point mutations in eukaryotic DNA.

2   A positive response in assays for mitotic recombination indicates the potential of a chemical to produce DNA interactions in a eukaryotic cell. The majority of such chemicals will be capable of producing either point mutations or chromosome aberrations in mammalian cells.

3. A positive response in assays for chromosome aneuploidy indicates the potential of a chemical to produce changes in chromosome number in eukaryotic

cells. However, in at least a proportion of such
chemicals, the effect may be specific for yeasts and
requires confirmation in a mammalian system.

Such a response should be reproducible in independent
experiments and should be significant when evaluated by an
appropriate statistical test. However, care should be taken
to ensure that the cultures used showed the "normal" levels of
spontaneous frequency for the event scored and that treatment
conditions were not such as to induce sporulation in
vegetative cultures. Considerably more weight can be placed
on results if an unambiguous dose response is observed, though
deviations from linearity are common for many of the genetic
end-points of yeast. There are no published data suggesting
that yeast assays produce false-positive results for any
consistent reason.

2.2.4.2 Negative results in yeast assays

Negative results may be obtained in yeast assays of
chemicals for genetic activity for a number of reasons:

(a) the test compound is inactive in eukaryotic cells;

(b) the compound has not been exposed to the appropriate
metabolic activation system;

(c) the relevant genetic end-point is not detectable in
yeast cultures, e.g., the induction of chromosome
aberrations; or

(d) the compound has not been tested over an appropriate
dose range, e.g., a fungicide may lead to cellular
toxicity before the genetically active cellular
concentrations are achieved. Another such example
may be found in assays such as those for chromosome
aneuploidy which frequently generate "humped"
dose-response curves where the genetically active
range requires the use of extensive concentration
ranges.

The validity of a negative result with a test chemical
will be of more general relevance if data are accompanied by
appropriate responses from positive control chemicals.

2.3   Unscheduled DNA Synthesis in Cultured Mammalian Cells

2.3.1   Introduction

The ability of living cells to remove damage induced in DNA was first reported in 1964 (Boyce & Howard-Flanders, 1964; Setlow & Carrier, 1964). It is now clear that cells can cut out portions of DNA damage in one strand of the double helix, replace the excised portion with undamaged DNA nucleotides by using the opposite strand as a template and rejoin the newly synthesized section to the pre-existing DNA strand (Hanawalt et al., 1979) (Fig. 2). This process is called excision repair and restores the original integrity of the DNA molecules.

Unscheduled DNA synthesis (UDS) is the term used to describe the synthesis of DNA during the excision repair of DNA damage and as such is distinct from the semiconservative replication that is confined to the "S" phase of the eukaryotic cell cycle. Rasmussen & Painter (1964) first reported the incorporation of ^{3}H thymidine into the DNA of cultured mammalian cells during the repair of damage induced by ultraviolet irradiation. These authors used autoradiography to detect UDS. This method involves culturing cells on glass slides, exposing them to a DNA-damaging agent in the presence of a medium containing high specific activity ^{3}H thymidine, and observing the radiolabel incorporated during UDS into cells that are not semiconservatively replicating DNA. This is done by way of an emulsion or film that detects the β emission from the tritium. The ability of substances to induce UDS in cultured cells is now widely used routinely to assess the genotoxic activity of compounds in mammalian systems. The assay is therefore a measure of the amount of repair produced and monitors neither the original lesion nor the consequences of repair. The amount of DNA replication associated with UDS is relatively low compared with the amount associated with semiconservative replication. If autoradiography is used to monitor this process, "S" phase cells that are undergoing semiconservative replication are readily eliminated from the analysis because of their heavy labelling indices. In this section, the measurement of radiolabelled thymidine incorporated during UDS by either autoradiography (Cleaver & Thomas, 1981) or liquid scintillation counting (LSC) will be considered (San & Stich, 1975; Martin et al., 1978). Unfortunately, the second method cannot distinguish between semiconservative and repair replication. It measures the total amount of DNA replication by monitoring the incorporation of ^{3}H thymidine into the total DNA, including cells that are actively replicating DNA semiconservatively. The elimination of the semiconservative

4

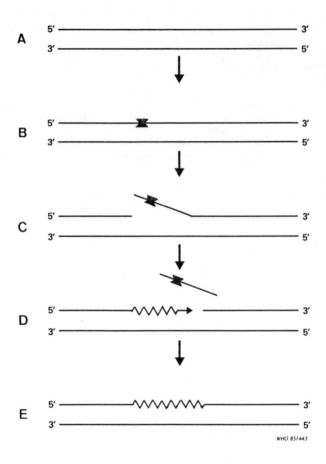

WHO 851443

Fig. 2.   A model of the excision repair of DNA: (A) represents a portion
of the DNA double helix from a mammalian cell. After exposure to
a genotoxic agent, DNA damage is induced in one of the strands
(B).   This   is   recognized   by   a   repair   endonuclease   which
introduces an incision in the phosphotriester backbone of the
strand containing the damage (C). An exonuclease cuts out the
portion of this strand containing the damage and resynthesis of
the resulting gap is begun by a DNA polymerase which uses the
opposite strand as a template (D). Resynthesis is completed and
the newly-made portion rejoined covalently to the existing strand
by a DNA ligase (E).   Thus, the initial integrity of the DNA
molecule is restored.

replicative process is therefore an essential prerequisite for this approach and can be achieved by various methods to be discussed later.

UDS has been detected in cells cultured from many mammalian species, in various cell types, and with different inducing agents. Human fibroblasts (San & Stich 1975) or human transformed cell lines such as HeLa (Martin et.al., 1978) are often used. One disadvantage of these cell lines is that they do not possess the ability to activate proximate carcinogens as does the liver in vivo, and thus additional metabolic activation in the form of a liver microsomal extract is required during chemical exposure. Alternative approaches to metabolic activation have been developed using epithelial cells derived from liver. These have been shown to retain some of the ability to activate proximate carcinogens (Williams, 1977; Dean & Hodson-Walker, 1979).

2.3.2   Chemical exposure and UDS

A large number of mutagens/carcinogens capable of inducing many types of DNA damage are known to induce UDS. The exact amount of this repair synthesis depends on (a) the particular mutagen/carcinogen in question, (b) the type of DNA repair process that operates on the damage induced, and (c) the size of the repair patch that is cut out to remove the damage prior to subsequent resynthesis. For example, it is known that some types of DNA damage, such as those induced by γ or X irradiation, are repaired relatively quickly in mammalian cells and involve the excision of only one to three bases per lesion (Regan & Setlow, 1974). Other types of damage such as UV radiation-induced pyrimidine dimers, are repaired more slowly and involve the replacement of from twenty to seventy bases per lesion (Regan & Setlow, 1974). The ability to detect UDS is further influenced by more obvious factors such as whether the cells used take up and incorporate (^{3}H)thymidine readily, the concentration and specific activity of the (^{3}H)thymidine, and the efficiency of the scintillation counter or film used to detect the radiolabel.

2.3.3   Procedure

2.3.3.1   The choice of a suitable cell line

Transformed cell lines, i.e., those possessing an infinite life ("immortal" cells) are preferred by some workers, but others have used primary cell lines with a finite life of some 30 - 40 generations. Generally, transformed cells (e.g., Hela) are easier to culture and grow more rapidly than primary cells. Rapid growth is an advantage for general cell culture, but it also means that the number of cells actively undertaking semi-conservative DNA replication in the population at a given time is higher, and the sensitivity of the assay is thus slightly reduced. This fact is less significant if autoradiography is used as the means of detecting UDS, since replicating "S" phase cells are readily excluded from cells at other stages of the cell cycle. However, if scintillation counting is used as the means of detecting UDS, precautions must be taken to greatly reduce the amount of semiconservative replication in the cell population. So far, it has not been possible to eliminate background levels of residual semiconservative replication entirely. In this respect, untransformed cell lines have a distinct advantage in that they stop dividing when they reach confluence because of contact inhibition when the amount of residual semiconservative DNA replication is considerably less than that seen in an actively dividing population.

A second important factor influencing the choice of cell line involves the activation of proximate carcinogens. Activation can be undertaken by the cell itself or by a microsomal liver extract added to the cell culture. The advantages of adding microsomal extract are that the same extract can be used in a range of other tests on different organisms, hence facilitating legitimate comparisons between various end-points. Furthermore, the source of extract can be easily varied if there is concern about the effects of a compound in a particular species, organ, or tissue. The major disadvantage is that certain concentrations of the extract iself can be toxic to some cell lines. The use of hepatocytes, because of their ability to activate proximate carcinogens without microsomal extract, would seem to offer a considerable advantage. However, a careful analysis of the hepatocyte line selected is essential prior to its use for the routine monitoring of DNA damaging agents, because it is also known that that such cells can exhibit a reduction in activation ability after a number of passages. Consequently, many research workers prefer to use freshly isolated primary hepatocytes for each experiment (Williams, 1977). Two further problems have been identified in the use of primary rat hepatocytes to screen chemicals for genotoxic activity (Lonati-Galligani et al., 1983). First, hepatocytes show a high cytoplasmic background labelling because of the incorporation of radioactive thymidine into mitochondrial DNA. Second, a large variation in the functional state of isolated hepatocytes affects the reproducibility of the system. Whatever cell type is chosen, it is imperative that a control chemical, known to require metabolic activation in order to induce DNA damage, is included in each experiment in order to monitor the activity of the endogenous metabolizing enzymes in that particular cell population.

For the autoradiography method, cells are cultured on cover slips or glass slides, and, for scintillation counting, the cells are cultured in disposable petri dishes.

2.3.4   The elimination of semiconservative replication

The minimizing of semiconservative DNA replication is an absolute prerequisite for the measurement of UDS by liquid scintillation counting. Although this is less important for autoradiography, some research workers prefer to suppress the semiconservative process in actively-dividing cells, especially if the percentage of such cells is high, and if long repair times are to be studied. In this last instance, the proportion of cells entering new rounds of DNA replication could be substantial.

Hydroxyurea, is commonly used at 10^{-3}M in UDS studies to suppress semi-conservative replication, and, at this dose, it has little effect on the amounts of UDS observed. It should be noted that this drug may react with the microsomal activation mixture to produce DNA damage (Andrae & Greim, 1979) and that, at high concentrations, inhibitory effects on DNA repair have been reported (Collins et al., 1977). Thus, unless its inclusion is essential, this drug is best avoided. When hydroxyurea is used, the appropriate controls to monitor possible effects such as reaction with microsomal extract to produce DNA damage should be undertaken. Additional treatments, such as incubation with medium containing low serum, or, as mentioned, growing cells to a monolayer are also used, as both approaches result in a cell population that contains considerably fewer replicating cells. Generally, when scintillation counting is the method selected for the detection of UDS, one or other of these two approaches is tried, before addition of hydroxyurea.

2.3.5   Chemical exposure

Prepared cultures are exposed to a range of doses of the chemical to be tested with, if required, the addition of microsomal extract and appropriate cofactors. The choice of a suitable dose range is governed by the toxicity of the compound. Studies should usually be undertaken at doses that induce 50% or less cytotoxicity as measured by, for example, Trypan Blue exclusion. In each experiment, it is imperative to include the appropriate control cultures to ensure that the system is functioning correctly. Thus, background UDS in untreated cells in the presence or absence of activation systems and solvents should be included as well as an

appropriate positive control known to be activated by the
microsomal activation system used (e.g., n-acetylamino-
fluorene). Cell cultures are usually exposed to five dose
levels of the test compound and, ideally, each dose is
duplicated. Exposure times are usually of the order of one to
a few hours, but longer periods have been studied.

2.3.6 Radiolabelling procedures

A typical procedure involves adding to the culture medium
(^{3}H)thymidine of a specific activity[a] greater than 20
Ci/mmol at 10 μCi/ml. This is usually carried out
immediately after the test compound is added so that both the
radiolabel and compound are present simultaneously for the
duration selected for the experiment.

2.3.7 Detection of UDS

The autoradiographic method involves the removal of the
medium containing the test compounds, followed by rinsing and
fixation of the cells, coating the slides with
autoradiographic emulsion and then drying them prior to
developing. Procedures will vary with the particular process
used and are described in detail by Cleaver & Thomas (1981).
After developing, the cells are stained and the grains in the
emulsion over the cell nuclei of control and treated samples
are either observed microscopically and counted visually or
with an electronic counter. The data are expressed as grains
per nucleus.

In the liquid scintillation method, culturing and exposure
procedures are similar to those for autoradiography, except
that more cells and more replicate samples are usually
analysed. The data are expressed as disintegrations per min
(dpm) of incorporated (^{3}H) thymidine per μg of DNA.
Hence, not only the amount of radioactivity per sample needs
to be determined, but also the amount of DNA. This can be
carried out by DNA extraction with perchloracetic acid
hydrolysis (Schmidt & Thannhauser, 1945), using one aliquot
for reaction with diphenylamine to measure DNA concentration
(Burton, 1956) and a second aliquot for scintillation counting
to measure (^{3}H) thymidine incorporation. Alternative
methods for estimating DNA concentrations are available (San &
Stich, 1975).

---

[a] The specific activity denotes how much of the thymidine is
actually radiolabelled.

2.3.8   Data processing and presentation

For a compound to be accepted as positive with the UDS
assay, there should be: (a) a dose-related increase in UDS,
and (b) a statistically-significant increase in UDS above that
of a negative control.   Data are usually presented as grain
counts   per   nucleus   (often   as   histograms),   or $\cdot(^3H)$
incorporation   as   dpm   per   μg   DNA,   as   determined   by
scintillation counting.   The data should include the results
from all treatments and controls.   At high concentrations of
test agents, the amounts of UDS may plateau because of the
saturation of repair mechanisms, or they may even decrease due
to cytotoxicity.   This again emphasises the importance of
undertaking experiments over a wide dose range, and then
selecting a narrow range from the initial data to verify a
potentially positive result.
Various criteria have been used for the definition of a
positive result.   Investigators have considered a compound
positive when it induced at least 150% of the control levels
of UDS as measured by liquid scintillation counting (San &
Stich, 1975), or when it induced at least 6 grains per nucleus
in excess of background levels with autoradiography (Williams,
1977).   In addition to such basic criteria, the data should
also be subjected to statistical analysis to determine whether
or not the increases are significant.   Cleaver & Thomas (1981)
recommend that, when 40 - 100 cells per slide are counted for
several slides per treatment, the average grain number for
each slide can be used as a measure of UDS, and the average
and standard error of these averages would be the more
suitable parameter for the amount and accuracy of the data.
When liquid scintillation counting is employed, the standard
deviation or standard error of the mean should be included to
describe the distribution of the data.   Additional analyses
such as analyses of variance, non parametric comparisons of
grain distribution, and estimates of the correlation between
UDS and dose can be undertaken, and the selection of the most
appropriate   method   will   depend   on   the   design   of   the
experiment.   The t-test, used by some, increases the chances
of obtaining false positives, whereas though the analysis of
variance   does   not   introduce   this   problem   it   does   reflect
cytotoxic   effects.   Ideally,   the   analysis   should   be
complemented with a contrast analysis that can distinguish
between treatments giving negative, positive, or cytotoxic
effects.   For a more complete review of the statistical
analysis of UDS data, the Gene-tox report on UDS tests by
Mitchell et al. (1983) can be referred to.

2.3.9   Discussion

UDS is a relatively straightforward approach for measuring
DNA repair and as such is extremely useful for examining
compounds that are potentially genotoxic for mammalian cells.
Nevertheless, it is usually undertaken as part of a battery of
screening tests. In exceptional cases, it may be the only
assay to provide a positive result and, in such cases, in vivo
tests should be undertaken to clarify this result. It should
also be noted that this assay detects the repair of DNA
damage. The assay would not detect a compound that induced an
unrepairable lesion in DNA, though the same compound would be
expected to induce genetic damage, e.g., mutations, in other
test systems. The usefulness of DNA repair assays in
screening is more fully reviewed by Cleaver (1982).

It is obvious from the procedural discussion in this
section that a number of different systems are currently used
to measure UDS. Thus, it would seem appropriate to list and
briefly evaluate critical factors that can influence each type
of assay, and which have been mentioned at various stages in
the text.

2.3.9.1 Choice of cell line

If possible, untransformed human fibroblasts or primary
rat hepatocytes should be used, because semiconservative DNA
replication is more readily suppressed in the former, whereas
the latter are essentially non-dividing and can themselves
activate proximate carcinogens. Furthermore, a relatively
large pre-existing data base is available for both cell types,
which enhances the possibility of making comparisons with
other compounds tested. However, it should be remembered that
primary rat hepatocytes exhibit high levels of incorporation
of radioactivity into the cytoplasm. It has been suggested
that for autoradiographic estimates, instead of subtracting
cytoplasmic grains from nuclear grains, as is usually done to
account for non-nuclear incorporation, grains overlying the
nucleus and a cytoplasmic area should be scored and plotted
separately in these cells (Lonati-Galliganai et al., 1983).
The variation in the functional state of freshly isolated
hepatocytes can be a problem and it is imperative to undertake
adequate controls to verify their ability to activate a
pro-carcinogen.

2.3.9.2 Choice of protocol

If rat hepatocytes are used, autoradiography is the method
of choice, as liquid scintillation counting (LSC) requires
such a large number of cells. Human fibroblasts can be

analysed either by autoradiography or by LSC, but it should be borne in mind that the latter approach requires more cells per sample, more duplicate samples, and the addition of hydroxyurea to supress residual semiconservative replication. At concentrations above 10^{-3} M, hydroxyurea can inhibit DNA repair and can also induce DNA damage by interacting with microsomal extract. These facts have to be considered when interpreting data. Where costs have to be kept to a minimum, it should be noted that a liquid scintillation counter is expensive compared with the cost of a microscope for autoradiography. However, a counter can process many samples automatically, whereas microscopic analysis is more time consuming.

2.3.9.3 Method of activating proximate carcinogens

The use of rat hepatocytes removes the necessity for the addition of microsomal extract. Whatever kind of microsomal activation is used, it is important to include appropriate controls to verify that the activation system is functional.

Finally, it should be emphasized that, regardless of the system used, the most important features in undertaking UDS studies are a full understanding of, and extensive experience with, the test system.

2.4 In Vitro Cytogenetics and Sister-Chromatid Exchange

2.4.1 Introduction

In vitro cytogenetic tests are designed to demonstrate the induction of chromosome damage (aberrations), visible under the light microscope, in cultured cells (Fig. 3). This usually involves examination at the metaphase stage of the cell cycle (Evans & O'Riordan, 1975; Savage, 1976). Though other methods such as anaphase analysis and enumeration of micronuclei have been used, they are not generally considered suitable for routine testing in cultured cells. A physical or chemical agent is classified as a clastogen if it produces an increase in the number of breaks in chromosomes over that found in control samples. Cytogenetic tests therefore assess gross damage to the DNA involving at least one double-strand break. A detailed discussion of the theoretical aspects of the development of chromosome aberrations is given in section 2.8.

Many agents only induce visible chromosome damage after the cells have undergone a round of DNA replication, and the test must be designed to allow enough time after treatment for aberrations to develop. However, damaged cells may not survive for more than one or two cell cycles after aberrations

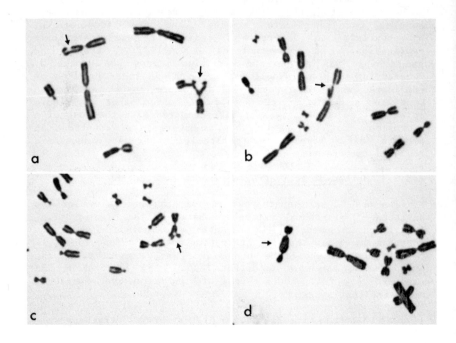

Fig. 3. Examples of chromosome aberrations in cultured Chinese hamster cells: (a) chromatid gap and interchange (incomplete); (b) chromatid break; (c) chromatid interchange; and (d) dicentric.

have been induced, and it is essential that cells should be examined in their first metaphase after treatment (Evans, 1976).

Induction of chromosome aberrations involves major damage to chromosome structure, and thus to the DNA, and so clastogenic agents must be viewed as potentially harmful. Although cells with visible chromosome aberrations are unlikely to have the potential to survive, repair of DNA damage may have occurred in apparently undamaged cells, and if this is error-prone, mutations could result. Certain types of chromosome damage, such as some deletions and rearrangements (translocations, inversions), may not be lethal. The comparatively high level of chromosomal disorders in man emphasizes the importance of chromosome changes in human populations (DHSS, 1982).

The preparation of material for examination of the chromosomes is technically simple, and this has undoubtedly contributed, in part, to the widespread use of short-term cytogenic tests. However, accurate and reliable scoring of metaphase chromosomes for aberrations does require a high level of expertise.

As its name implies, sister chromatid exchange (SCE) involves an apparently symmetrical change between chromatids within a chromosome (i.e., between identical sequences of DNA). SCEs are only visible under the microscope if sister chromatids can be distinguished (Fig. 4); this requires different culture methods from those used in the preparation of metaphases for the scoring of chromosome aberrations. Because of the ease of preparation and scoring, it is a very widely-used test in the study of mutagens. SCE induction alone is not generally accepted as sufficient evidence to classify an agent as mutagenic. The mechanism of SCE induction is not fully understood, though a number of models have been proposed (Wolff, 1982). Some clastogens induce only a small, or no, increase in SCEs, X-irradiation being a particularly striking example. There is a high background level of SCE compared with chromosome aberrations; it is rare to find many cells without SCEs in untreated samples. This may be partly due to the 5-bromodeoxyuridine (BrdUrd) that is added to the culture medium in order to visualise SCEs, since BrdUrd itself is known to induce SCEs (Latt et al., 1981). This basal level also implies that cells with SCEs are capable of subsequent growth. SCE evaluation may thus be a more valid indicator than chromosome breakage of events compatible with cell survival, hence its widespread use in mutagenicity screening programmes.

2.4.2   Procedure: chromosomal aberrations

The techniques used in the study of chromosomal aberration have been described in detail by Evans (1976) and in the Gene-Tox reports of Latt et al. (1981) and Preston et al. (1981).

2.4.2.1 Cell types

Two types of cells are used most widely for both tests. These are CHO, an established fibroblast cell line, derived from Chinese hamster ovary, and human peripheral blood lymphocytes (mononuclear white blood cells). The small number of chromosomes in CHO cells (modal number 22) makes scoring relatively straight forward. It is an easy cell line to maintain, using standard tissue culture techniques, and, with

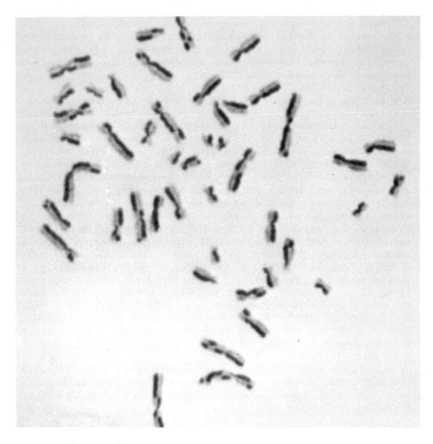

Fig. 4. Sister chromatid exchanges in human lymphocytes.

a cell cycle time of 12 - 14 h, grows very rapidly (Latt et al., 1981; Preston et al., 1981; Dean & Danford, 1985).

Human peripheral lymphocytes do not divide spontaneously in culture, but can be stimulated to divide by treatment with a mitogen such as phytohaemagglutinin (PHA). Cultures are initiated from fresh blood samples and are not maintained for more than a few cell divisions. The first metaphase after the addition of the mitogen is not reached for about 36 - 40 h, after which the cells divide about every 18 h, with considerable variation, both within and between cultures. Culture methods are described in detail by Dean & Danford (1975) and Evans & O'Riordan (1975).

Other cell lines have been used in cytogenetic assays, for example, lines with endogenous metabolizing capacity, such as rat liver epithelial cells (Dean & Hodson-Walker, 1979). It is important for a cell line to be fully validated with a range of suitable chemicals before being used for routine testing.

Initially, information on the toxicity of a test agent is required, and subsequently, concentrations up to a level where some toxicity is observed are used in the cytogenetic assay. Toxicity can be assessed, for example, by measurement of the mitotic index or by cell counts. To obtain sufficient data from the chromosomal aberration assay, a minimum of 3 replicate cultures of each of 3 doses, or 2 replicates of 4 doses is advisable, in addition to a negative control (solvent only) and a positive control. With lymphocyte cultures, it is recommended to use blood from at least two different donors in each experiment. Under rare circumstances, it may be possible to use a positive control structurally related to the test material; more commonly, the positive control will be a known clastogen. A direct-acting clastogen or one requiring metabolic activation is used, as appropriate (see below). The doses of the test agent should range from a concentration showing some toxicity down to 1/4 or 1/8 of this, or equivalent log doses. Since many clastogens only show effects close to the toxic dose, there is rarely any advantage in selecting lower concentrations for routine screening.

2.4.2.2 Culture methods

Cell lines are grown either in small tissue-culture flasks or directly on sterile microscopic slides or cover slips until the cells are proliferating. The agent under study is then introduced, preferably by replacing the culture medium with medium plus agent. Lymphocytes do not attach to culture flasks or slides, and are usually grown in small bottles as suspension cultures. The test agent can be added to lymphocyte cultures when they are set up. It is preferable, however, to allow time for the cells to leave the G_0 stage before adding the test agent, because toxic concentrations of the test agent may prevent the cells from entering the cell cycle. Thus, addition of the test agent after 24 - 36 h of culture is more likely to be effective.

Modifications to either system may be required; for example, volatile or gaseous compounds should be tested in a closed system. In some instances, components in the serum used in the culture medium may bind to the test agent, in which case it is desirable to treat the cells in serum-free medium for a few hours, and then continue culturing in normal medium. Erythrocytes (red blood cells), present in lymphocyte cultures set up from whole blood, can also bind the test agent. Various methods of separating out the lymphocytes are available (Boyum, 1968), though whole blood cultures are more widely used. Unless the cell line has been shown to have intrinsic metabolizing capabilities, or there is strong evidence that the agent under test is direct-acting (requiring no metabolism), a metabolizing system, such as an S9 microsome fraction obtained from rat liver, must be included (section 2.1). When testing chemicals of unknown mutagenic activity, assays both with and without a metabolizing system are required. If there is compelling evidence that the agent is either direct-acting or requires activation, then the first test can be carried out either without or with a metabolizing system. If equivocal or negative results are obtained, further tests will be necessary.

The times of exposure differ between the two test systems, and are detailed below, but it is important to bear in mind that S9 can be toxic to mammalian cells. Thus the time of exposure to the test agent may be limited to only 1/2 - 3 h in assays using S9. In these cases, the medium containing the test material and S9 is replaced by normal medium, until the cells are harvested. Treatment at toxic doses may extend the cell cycle time, and the period between treatment with the test chemical and harvesting should be extended accordingly. It may be necessary to use more than one sampling time; this is discussed in more detail in section 2.4.5.

2.4.2.3 Chromosome assay

Following the introduction of the test agent, the cells are incubated for between one and two cell cycles so that the majority of the mitotic cells are in the first metaphase after treatment, when harvested. Before harvesting, a spindle poison such as colchicine is added to arrest cells at metaphase. The cells are treated with a hypotonic solution, such as 0.56% (0.075 M) potassium chloride, and then fixed, usually with a freshly prepared 3:1 mixture of methanol and glacial acetic acid. Subsequently, the cells are stained with Giemsa, orcein, or other chromosome stain, and are then examined under the microscope. The slides should be coded randomly and independently, and at least 100 metaphases scored from each replicate. However, if the mitotic index is greatly reduced at the highest dose, it is not always possible to score 100 cells. Aberration types are usually classified into chromatid (involving only one chromatid) and chromosomal or isochromatid (affecting both chromatids) and are clearly described by Evans & O'Riordan (1975), Savage (1976), ISCN (1978), and Scott et al. (1983). Other classification systems have been devised, such as that of Buckton et al. (1962), in which chromosome aberrations are classified as stable (C_s), such as translocations, or unstable (C_u), such as dicentrics, depending on whether or not they can be maintained through successive cell cycles. Banding techniques (Evans, 1976), commonly used for detailed chromosome analysis, are rarely used for routine screening.

2.4.3 Procedure: sister chromatid exchange

Cultures to demonstrate SCEs are set up as for chromosome assays, but in addition to the test agent, BrdUrd is present, at concentrations of 10 - 25 µM, throughout the period from treatment to harvesting. The cells must be allowed to pass through two rounds of DNA replication (S-phases) before harvesting. BrdUrd is incorporated into the newly synthesized DNA in place of thymidine, and thus, at the first metaphase, all chromatids possess one DNA strand containing BUdR and one containing thymidine. The chromatids separate at anaphase, and at the second S-phase, the DNA synthesized again contains BUdR. Since one DNA template is unsubstituted and the other substituted with BUdR, the chromosomes now contain DNA with one chromatid completely (bifiliarly) substituted and the other, half (unifiliarly) substituted with BrdUrd. These chromatids stain differentially following the treatment described below.

The cultures are harvested as usual but, thereafter, stained with Hoechst 33258 solution, exposed to a light source emitting long-wave UV radiation, and then stained with Giemsa. The bifiliarly substituted chromatids stain to a much lesser degree than the unifiliarly substituted chromatids. Where SCE has occurred, a change in the staining intensity can be seen on one chromatid, with a reciprocal change on the other (Perry & Wolff, 1974). These second metaphase chromosomes are referred to as harlequin chromosomes. First metaphase cells have uniformly darkly stained chromatids, and third and subsequent metaphases have a mixture of pale-staining and harlequin chromosomes. Since second division metaphases can be recognized by having entirely harlequin chromosomes, the problem of mitotic delay is not so great with SCE analysis as with assessment of chromosome aberrations. Though there may be a reduction in the proportion of second-division metaphases at the highest doses, these can be recognized and scored. A number of reviews of SCEs are available; Latt et al. (1977), Perry (1980), and Wolff (1982) include photographs of differentially stained chromosomes.

The slides should also be coded, and at least 30 (preferably 50 or more) metaphases examined from each culture.

2.4.4   Procedure: scoring

Accurate identification of chromosome aberrations and scoring of SCEs requires a high degree of skill, and should only be undertaken by suitably trained and experienced personnel. Descriptions of aberrations do not usually include details of potential artefacts, and it is essential to appreciate that there are a number of normal chromosome orientations which the inexperienced may score as aberrations. In addition, the quality of the material must be sufficiently high for accurate assessment, and analysis of "fuzzy", overlapping, or highly-scattered chromosomes should not be attempted.

Results, including types of aberrations observed, should be recorded on a suitable score-sheet. For chromosome aberrations, some record, either the vernier reading on the microscope stage or a photograph of each aberrant cells, is usually taken. It is obviously important to ensure that the same metaphases are not scored twice. For further details, see section 2.8.

2.4.5   Extent of testing

The decision as to whether a chemical has been tested sufficiently to classify it as positive or negative in these test systems is not always clear cut. If a clear positive response is seen, or if there is no increase above negative control levels at any dose, provided there is evidence of toxicity at the highest dose, no further testing is necessary. If, however, the negative control gives unusually high values, or the positive control fails to induce the expected number of aberrations, this would suggest that the experiment should be repeated. A weakly positive response will often need to be confirmed in an additional experiment, though, under some circumstances, adequate data may be obtained from simply scoring additional metaphases on slides already examined. Otherwise, it may be necessary to repeat the experiment, either exactly as before or using different dose levels or exposure times. A particularly important aspect of cell kinetics under the influence of toxic doses is the delay in the cell cycle time. Thus, an apparently negative dose-response can be obtained if cells at higher doses have not undergone a round of DNA replication between treatment and harvesting, when examining an S-dependent agent. In these cases, a later sampling time is required in a repeat experiment.

2.4.6   Data processing and presentation

When a clear dose-related increase in chromosomal aberrations is obtained, or when there is clearly no increase above control levels, the result may be obvious without the need for statistical analysis. It is, however, always advisable that results should be subjected to an appropriate statistical analysis. Metaphase analysis, particularly if gaps are excluded, can yield such small numbers of aberrations that objective interpretation is only feasible after such statistical tests as the Chi^2 and Fisher's Exact test (Sokal & Rohlf, 1969).

The data are best presented in tabular form showing the results for each dose, and the positive and negative controls, and including details of the cell line, culture conditions, and slide codes. The minimum data required are: the doses, number of metaphases observed from each culture, and either the percentage of aberrant metaphases, including and excluding gaps, and the total number of aberrations, or the average number of SCEs per cell. Further breakdown of chromosomal aberrations into chromatid/chromosomal-type aberrations, and classes within these groups (gaps, breaks, exchanges, etc.) is also essential. Graphic representation of a dose-response can also be helpful.

Test agents are regarded as unequivocably positive if a dose-related increase is observed over 3 or 4 doses (including the negative control), and/or 3 or 4 doses give aberration or SCE levels significantly higher than the negative control level. If no dose-related increase is observed, and no dose gives a significantly higher frequency of chromosome aberrations or SCEs than the control, then the data are interpreted as negative. Weak or marginal findings usually require additional data or testing, but a reproducible dose response rising just above control levels, provided this is statistically significant, is the criterion for the designation of a weakly positive result.

Compounds should normally be tested up to concentrations that induce detectable toxicity or reduction in mitotic index. Agents that show no evidence of toxicity in preliminary studies should be tested to the limit of solubility. However, very high concentrations of some non-toxic chemicals may interfere with culture conditions, and the maximum dose level should be decided on a case by case basis.

Occasionally, a single high value is found at one dose or replicate culture. This requires a repeat experiment, using a narrower dose range above and below that dose. If the increase in aberrations or SCEs at the dose is not reproduced, then the isolated result can be discounted. Another potential problem of interpretation is an increase in chromatid gaps at the highest dose. The significance of gaps is discussed in section 2.8. In the absence of an increase in other types of aberrations, it is possible that the increase in gaps is associated with the cytotoxicity of the test material and is not necessarily of genotoxic significance. In such instances, it is particularly important to consider data from other test systems before evaluating the mutagenicity of the chemical.

2.4.7   Discussion

2.4.7.1   Critical factors

The assessment of cytogenetic damage and SCEs depends crucially on accurate scoring. It must be emphasized that this, in turn, depends on the training and experience of the scorer as well as the quality of the material. Both under- and over-estimation can result from failure to meet these criteria.

It is also necessary for the cell line used to be suitably validated with known clastogens before it is used routinely. Even where an apparently strongly positive response is obtained, the results may be viewed with question if, for example, a highly unstable cell line is used. This emphasizes the need to use either the standard cell types (CHO or lymphocytes) or to establish an adequate data base for a new cell line, particularly with regard to its metabolizing capacity and the level of aberrations in untreated cells.

2.4.7.2   Experimental design and analysis

If information is available on the chemical structure and metabolizing requirements of the test agent, the most suitable medium for treating the cells (complete or serum-free) can be assessed. The value of using toxic doses is emphasised in cases where serum components are suspected to react with the test agent, as it serves to confirm that the agent has entered the cells.

A particularly important aspect is the influence of the test agent on the cell cycle time. Mitotic delay is frequently found at toxic doses, and this may result in the examination of metaphases in which visible aberrations have not had time to develop. However, the next lowest dose should indicate whether or not this is the case; this can be further checked by testing additional doses and sampling times. With SCEs, the problem still arises, but because second division metaphases can be recognised and are scored, it is possible to assess whether or not significant mitotic delay has occurred.

The system used to ensure that metabolic activation has occurred can lead to a number of problems. The toxicity of S9 has already been mentioned, and cells retaining metabolic activation may vary in the extent and range of activation, and, furthermore, some may lose their activating ability following repeated subculturing. A positive control structurally related to the test compound, in addition to a standard positive control, is ideal, but in practice this is rarely available.

An assessment of clastogenicity can only be accepted if the results from negative and positive controls are within the expected range. The occurrence of a high value in the negative control cultures is by no means unusual, but, in a well-characterized line, its validity can be tested statistically. Any indication that a positive control agent (especially one requiring activation) has not been detected would also require a repeat of the experiment.

Further studies are necessary to clarify unexpected or ambiguous results, in which case the use of additional sampling times will often provide confirmatory data. If a clear negative or positive result is obtained, there is usually no need for verification in a second experiment. If toxic doses cannot be achieved, a different solvent or a variation in the exposure time should be considered. Unfortunately, the low tolerance of cultured mammalian cells to pH changes and organic solvents precludes more than slight variations in the culture conditions.

2.4.8   Conclusions

The ability of a chemical to produce undoubted double-strand breaks, i.e., a strong clastogenic action, is an important finding as is strong evidence that there is no such activity. Thus, it is important to try to resolve the ambiguous and weakly positive results. These can usually be clarified by further testing. An increase in gaps alone only implies a discontinuity in staining, and therefore may not be due to double-strand breaks. Agents that induce gaps may cause disturbances in normal chromosome structure, but not necessarily chromosome breakage (section 2.8). Since the precise mechanism of SCE induction is not fully understood, the genetic significance of SCEs cannot be determined, at present. However, they reflect a direct interaction of chemicals with DNA and represent a useful system for the detecion of genotoxic chemicals. With certain exceptions, chromosome-aberration and SCE assays correlate well with other tests.

2.5   In Vitro Cell-Mutation Assays

2.5.1   Principles and scientific basis of the assay

The use of cultured mammalian cells, including human cells, for mutation studies can give a measure of the intrinsic response of the mammalian genome and its maintenance processes to mutagens, while offering rapidity of assay and ease of treatment compared with the use of whole animals.

Several forward and reverse mutation selection systems are available for use with cultured cells (Abbondandolo, 1977). The basis of the majority is that the cells are cultured in a "selective medium" containing a toxic compound or anti-metabolite (called the "selective agent") which is toxic to all normal, non-mutant cells, but in which rare, mutant cells can continue to grow to form colonies. A major requirement for such assays is that evidence should be provided that the end-point of the measurement is a mutational event that occurs at a specific gene locus, that is, it should be consistent with the induction of a heritable alteration in the DNA sequence. In general, detailed biochemical analysis of the gene product and cytogenetic study of the chromosomes points to the mutational origin of the selected colonies, though it is possible that some of the phenotypic changes observed may be the result of the kinds of non-mutational changes in gene expression that occur during normal development ("epigenetic events") (Siminovitch, 1976).

One problem associated with the selection of mutants of mammalian cells is that two copies of each gene are present in a normal diploid cell, and, in many cases, the mutant gene product acts recessively: that is, adequate gene product is transcribed from one (non-mutant) gene copy to fulfil the cell's needs. In this case, mutation of both genes in a diploid cell (a very rare event) is necessary to detect the mutant phenotype. Therefore, mutation of such genes in cultured mammalian cells is studied in the hemizygous or heterozygous state, using either X-chromosome genes (where only one X is present in male cells, or only one active X in female cells) or autosomal genes that have either been found, or deliberately selected to be hemizygous in some cells lines.

An example of an X-chromosome-located gene that is the basis of a mutation selection system is the gene coding for the enzyme hypoxanthine-guanine phosphoribosyltransferase (HPRT). HPRT is one of a number of "salvage" enzymes in which the function is to salvage the degradation products of nucleic acid synthesis (purines and pyrimidines), but which are not essential for the survival of the cultured cells, since these bases can be synthesized de novo. HPRT catalyses the conversion of guanine and hypoxanthine to the corresponding nucleoside-5'-monophosphates. In cells containing HPRT, toxic purine analogues, for example 6-thioguanine or 8-azaguanine, are also incorporated, and this forms the basis of the selection of mutants. Thus, cells with normal, non-mutant HPRT are killed when they are cultured in the presence of these selective agents, but mutants, with altered, or non-functional HPRT (or its complete absence) are able to survive and form colonies, because the toxic analogues are not incorporated into DNA or RNA. Purines continue to be made in the mutant cells by the de novo pathway. It is interesting to note that human beings with a rare sex-linked recessive disease, the Lesch-Nyhan syndrome, are mutant at the HPRT locus. All cells from males with this disorder are HPRT deficient and are resistant to the toxic effects of 6-thioguanine and 8-azaguanine.

Another gene coding for a "salvage" enzyme, this time on an autosomal chromosome, is the thymidine kinase (TK) gene. This enzyme incorporates exogenously supplied thymidine, and its toxic analogues, into the cell. In this case, both homozygous ($TK^+/+$) and heterozygous ($TK^+/1$) diploid cells contain sufficient thymidine kinase for the cells to be killed when they are cultured in the presence of toxic pyrimidine base analogues such as 5-bromodeoxyuridine or trifluorothymidine. Mutants that do not contain any functional TK ($TK^-/-$) do not incorporate the analogues, and are therefore able to survive and form colonies in the presence of these selective agents. Normal diploid cells contain two copies of the TK gene, and as simultaneous mutation of both genes is a very rare event, a heterozygous($TK^+/-$) cell line must first be constructed for mutation assays based on this enzyme to be possible.

Since complete loss of the "salvage" enzymes HPRT and TK is not deleterious to cultured mammalian cells, all types of mutations, including base-pair substitution (which may result in altered gene product), frame-shifts, and deletions (which result in complete lack of enzyme) should be detected. Evidence to support this has been presented in the considerable literature available on the HPRT locus (Caskey & Krush, 1979) and the TK locus (Hozier et al., 1981).

In both the above cases, the mutant gene product acts recessively. A few mutation systems rely on the semi-dominant action of the mutant gene product, and in these cases mutation in only one of the two genes present in a diploid cell is necessary to detect the mutant phenotype. For example, mutation to the semi-dominant phenotype of ouabain-resistance involves an essential enzyme, the membrane-bound Na^+/K^+-dependent ATPase (Baker et al., 1974). Ouabain kills cells by binding to this enzyme and causing an imbalance in ion flow, but rare mutants can be found that fail to bind

ouabain while retaining functional ATPase activity. The range
of mutations detected by ouabain resistance would be expected
to be much more restricted than for the non-essential salvage
enzymes, because, if a large mutagenic change, e.g., a
deletion, occurred in the gene coding for the Na^+/K^+
ATPase, the essential enzyme function would be lost together
with ouabain binding, and the mutant cell would die. Some
evidence has been presented to support this conclusion (Baker,
1979).

2.5.2   Relevance and limitations

In the testing of potential chemical mutagens, a major
limitation of cultured mammalian cell systems is the
difficulty of simulating in vitro the type and quantity of
metabolic activation that may occur in different tissues in
vivo. This is because the cultured cells lack the full range
of enzymes required to activate the diverse range of potential
mutagens and carcinogens encountered in the environment.
Thus, the experiments must be conducted in the presence of an
"exogenous" metabolic activation system. This may be supplied
by the use of rat liver homogenates ('S9') or by
co-cultivating the tester cells with metabolically competent
cells, such as freshly isolated rat hepatocytes. The choice
of the metabolizing system(s) and the way that it is applied
in the assay has great importance for the efficiency of the
test in predicting the mutagenic or carcinogenic potential of
chemicals that require activation. Considerable further work
is required to determine the optimal conditions for the in
vitro activation of many chemicals.

2.5.3   Procedure

2.5.3.1 Outline of the basic technique

A large population of cells is exposed to the test
substance, with and without an exogenous metabolic activation
system, for a defined period of time. After removal of the
test substance, the cytotoxicity is determined by measuring
the colony-forming ability and/or the growth rate of the
cultures after treatment. Bulk cultures of the treated cells
are maintained in a growth medium for a sufficient period of
time to allow the newly induced mutations to be detected.
During this period, known as the expression time, the growth
rate can be monitored and the cells sub-cultured if
necessary. The mutant frequency is then determined by seeding
known numbers of cells at high density in a medium containing
a selective agent to detect the number of mutant colonies, and
at a lower density in a medium without selection to determine

the cloning efficiency. After a suitable incubation time, colonies are counted. The mutant frequency per viable cell is derived by adjusting the number of mutant colonies in the selective medium by the estimate of viable, colony-forming cells obtained from the number of colonies in the non-selective medium.

Calculations

Cloning efficiency (CE)

Mean colonies per plate in non-selective medium
$$\frac{\text{Mean colonies per plate in non-selective medium}}{\text{Total cells seeded per plate in non-selective medium}}$$

Mutant frequency (ME)

$$\frac{\text{Mean mutant colonies per plate in selective medium}}{\text{Total cells seeded per plate in selective medium}}$$

Mutant frequency per survivor $= \dfrac{MF}{CE}$

Each experiment contains "control" (untreated) cultures so that the background (spontaneous) mutant frequency can be determined.

2.5.3.2 Cell types and selective systems

Many different cell types, including cells of human, rat, mouse, and hamster origin, and a wide variety of selective systems are available for potential gene mutation assay (Abbondandolo, 1977; Holstein et al., 1979). Many of these fulfil the criteria suggested for the use of mammalian cells in such assays, for example, a sound genetic basis for the system, high cloning efficiency, low spontaneous mutation frequency, and a demonstrated sensitivity to a variety of chemical mutagens. However, in practice, only three cell lines, the V79 and CHO Chinese hamster-derived cell lines, and L4178Y mouse lymphoma cells have been widely used for large-scale mammalian cell in vitro assays. In all three cases, HPRT and the Na+/K+ ATPase genes have been used as the genetic systems for the basis of mutant selection. In addition, an L5178Y cell line, heterozygous at the TK locus (L5178Y TK^{+}/-), has been developed by Clive and co-workers (Clive et al., 1972), and has been extensively used for the selection of TK mutants in mutation assays. More recently, a

CHO cell line, heterozygous at the TK locus, has also been developed (Adair et al., 1980). Several reviews are available which discuss the general principles of mammalian cell assays (Hsie et al., 1979; Fox, 1981) and the V79 (Bradley et al., 1981), CHO (Hsie et al., 1981), and L5178Y (Clive et al., 1983) cell lines, in particular. Many of the critical factors involved are discussed in these papers and the extensive available literature is cited. Considerable variations exist in the protocols for mutation assays using different mammalian cell lines and selective systems. These should be carefully studied, preferably in close consultation with experienced investigators in this field.

Some of the problems associated with this assay have been highlighted and discussed in the recently conducted collaborative study on short-term in vitro tests, by Ashby et al. (1985), and some recommendations for future improvements have been made.

2.5.3.3 Culture conditions

Culture conditions should be well-defined, and the cells should be maintained under optimal growth conditions throughout the experiment. Cultured cells require the presence of serum to maintain growth, and the serum batch may affect growth rate, cloning efficiency, and mutant frequency. Batches of serum should therefore be carefully pretested and a large volume of a suitable batch stored frozen. Medium, pH, temperature, humidity, and cell dispersion techniques are among the critical factors in mammalian cell culture techniques and should be carefully controlled if reproducible data are to be obtained.

2.5.3.4 Treatment

To ensure that all stages of the cell cycle are exposed to the test substance, exponentially growing cells in tissue culture medium should normally be used. Great care should be taken to standardize the treatment conditions. Medium, pH, serum content, incubation conditions, and cell density during treatment should all be carefully controlled. The cultures should be protected from light during treatment, and suspension cultures should be shaken. The test substance should be dissolved just before use, preferably in tissue culture medium. Other vehicles may be used, for example, dimethyl sulfoxide, but each should be tested to be certain that its presence has no effect on cell viability or growth rate. For initial toxicity studies, a wide range of molarity of the test substance should be used. When the toxic response has been determined, the mutation experiment should cover several concentrations (usually a minimum of four) ranging from non-toxic (90 - 100% survival of the treated cells) to toxic (1 - 10% survival). Greater levels of kill are not recommended (Bradley et al., 1981). Treatment time is generally for 1 - 5 h, although 16 h (Bradley et al., 1981) or longer may be appropriate (Cole et al., 1982).

2.5.3.5 Expression time

After the cells have been exposed to a mutagen, they must be cultured in a non-selective medium for a period of time so that (a) the mutagen-induced damage can be "fixed" in the DNA, and (b) the constitutive level of the non-mutant enzyme, and its mRNA, can decrease to a negligible level. The time required for a new mutation to be phenotypically expressed as a mutant enzyme (the "phenotypic expression period") will depend on the initial number of non-mutant enzyme (and mRNA) molecules, their half life under physiological conditions, and the rate of cell division. The expression time varies with the cell line, the selective system, and possibly also the mutagen treatment. After the maximum induced mutant frequency has been observed, there may be a plateau in the frequency of mutants, while in other cases, there may be a peak in the number of mutants followed by a fall in the frequency. For example, it has been found that induced ouabain-resistant mutants are first observed within 24 h of mutagen treatment, reach a maximum 48 - 72 h after treatment, and later remain at an approximately constant value. The thioguanine-resistant phenotype, however, requires a minimum of 6 - 7 days after treatment before new mutations are fully expressed, after which there is again a plateau in the mutant frequency. In contrast to these observations, mutations at the TK locus reach a peak value 48 - 72 h after treatment, and then there is a marked decline in frequency with time. For quantitative mutation studies, it is very important that near-optimal phenotypic expression of induced mutation should be observed, and the shape of the expression time curve for newly-induced mutants must be carefully determined by experiment by each laboratory, under well-defined conditions, using a number of different mutagens.

2.5.3.6 Choice and concentration of selective agent

The concentration of the selective agent is one of the most critical factors (Thompson & Baker, 1973). The dose should be high enough for complete kill of non-mutant cells and the mutant frequency at the chosen concentration should not be affected by small variations that may occur in day-to-day culture conditions. 6-Thioguanine is generally considered to be a more stringent selective agent for the selection of HPRT mutants than 8-azaguanine, and is the agent of choice for mouse cells, as azaguanine is non-toxic to these cells. Trifluorothymidine, which is recommended for the selection of TK mutants, is both heat and light unstable and must be handled with great care.

2.5.3.7 Stability of the spontaneous mutant frequency

A high and variable spontaneous mutant frequency can cause considerable problems with data interpretation. Several methods are available for maintaining a low, stable frequency:

(a) The cell line can be re-cloned to establish a suitable sub-line. A large frozen stock can then be stored in liquid nitrogen and one vial used for each experiment.

(b) Cells regularly sub-cultured to maintain stocks should be diluted to low density to remove pre-existing mutants.

(c) For the TK and HPRT systems, pre-existing mutants lacking these enzymes can be removed from the population by growing the cells in medium containing aminopterin. This anti-metabolite blocks the de novo purine and pyrimidine synthesis pathways. If thymidine and hypoxanthine are also added to the medium (called "HAT" medium), non-mutant cells containing TK and HPRT continue to grow using the "salvage" pathway. Mutant TK⁻ or HPRT⁻ cells die in HAT medium, because they are unable to use either the de novo or the "salvage" pathways for nucleotide synthesis. After "HAT" treatment, again, a large stock of cells can be stored in liquid nitrogen for future use.

2.5.3.8 Provision for metabolic conversion

Three methods of supplying exogenous mammalian activation systems are available (Bartsch et al., 1982).

(a) Rodent liver preparations ("S9") (see also section above)

These can be prepared from untreated animals (usually rats) or from animals pre-treated with "inducing agent" (e.g., phenobarbital, 3-methylcholanthrene, or Aroclor® 1254) to induce high levels of the mixed-function oxidases that catalyse the metabolic activation steps. Such preparations have been widely used with mammalian cells (Kuroki et al., 1977, 1979; Bartsch et al., 1979; Clive et al., 1979; Amacher

& Turner, 1981, 1982a,b). These papers contain detailed methods for the preparation of both S9 and the NADPH energy generating systems ("co-factor mix") for use with mammalian cell cultures.

A batch of S9 should be prepared, tested for sterility, and stored for up to 3 months at -70 °C, or in liquid nitrogen. Both S9 and the co-factor mix should only be thawed immediately before use.

(b) Cell-mediated metabolism

In this case, the indicator cells (e.g., L5178Y or V79) are co-cultivated with metabolically-competent cells, e.g., freshly-isolated rat hepatocytes (Amacher & Paillet, 1983) or hamster cell lines such as BHK or SHE (Langenbach et al., 1981; Bartsch et al, 1982). The pro-mutagen or -carcinogen is metabolized to the active product by the competent cells and diffuses into the indicator cells, where it reacts with the DNA.

(c) The host-mediated assay

Finally, the cultured cells may be placed inside the body of an animal (usually a mouse) which is treated with the test substance. After a suitable period, the cells are withdrawn, and the mutant frequency determined. For example, L5178Y cells can be grown in the peritoneal cavity of compatible mice (Fischer et al., 1974) or V79 cells in diffusion chambers in mice (Sirianni et al., 1979).

2.5.3.9 Controls and internal monitoring

For each experiment, positive and negative controls are required. A negative control is necessary to check the background mutant frequency. It should consist of no treatment and/or the solvent as used to dissolve the test substance. Two separate positive controls (to check that the assay is performing correctly) are necessary, one of which should require metabolic activation. It is an advantage if a positive control with a known dose-response is used, so that the sensitivity of the assay can be assessed in each experiment.

Cell cultures should be periodically checked for mycoplasma contamination (Russel et al., 1975) and can be periodically karyotyped to check chromosome stability.

2.5.3.10 Population size, replicates, and reproducibility

(a) Population size

The power and sensitivity of the test should be pre-determined, taking the toxic effect of the test substance and the mutant frequency in the untreated population into account. The number of cells to be treated, sub-cultured, and exposed to selection should be sufficient for a particular increase over the control mean to be detected. The precise numbers depend on the cell line and selective system, but as a general guide it has been suggested that ten times the inverse of the spontaneous mutant frequency should be used. This means, for example, that if the spontaneous mutant frequency is 1×10^{-6}, then 10^7 visible cells should be used for each treatment level. If there is substantial initial toxicity, this number should be increased correspondingly. Similar care should be taken over the numbers of cells sub-cultured during the expression period, to avoid sampling error. The number of cells exposed to selection should be such that the numbers of mutant colonies observed on both control and test plates are sufficient for statistical analysis.

(b) Replication

One protocol recommends that duplicate samples should be treated, sub-cultured, and plated in every experiment (Clive et al., 1979). Alternatively, single very large populations can be used for each treatment level.

(c) Reproducibility

The determinations should be quantitative and reproducible. The whole experiment should be carried out at least twice using freshly prepared test substance, though not necessarily over precisely the same dose range. If both experiments give a positive or negative result, this could be considered acceptable. However, for low or equivocal responses, further experimentation may be necessary.

2.5.4 Data processing and presentation

2.5.4.1 Treatment of results

The test report should include precise details of all methods used in the test procedure. All validation data should be provided and retained for further reference.

Data should be presented in tabular form. All original data, including toxicity data, absolute cloning efficiency of the control cultures, and individual colony counts for the treated and control groups should be presented for both mutation induction and survival plates. Survival and cloning efficiencies should be presented as a percentage of the controls. Mutant frequency should be presented as per 10^6 clonable cells. Possible toxicity of the vehicle should be indicated.

2.5.4.2 Evaluation of results

Several criteria have been suggested for determining a positive result, one of which is a statistically significant, concentration-related increase in the mutant frequency. An alternative is based on the detection of a reproducible and statistically significant positive response for at least one concentration of the test substance. The problem with such an approach is that, although several methods of statistical analysis have been published (Clive et al., 1979; Amacher & Turner, 1981; Snee & Irr, 1981; Tan & Hsie, 1981), there is, at present, no general concensus as to the most appropriate method. Further work is required on the optimum experimental design and statistical analysis of mammalian cell assays.

A substance that does not produce either a reproducible concentration-related increase in mutant frequency or a reproducible significant positive result at any one test point is considered non-mutagenic in this test.

2.5.4.3 Ambiguous results

Ideally, experimental design should be such that ambiguous results do not occur. Examples of ambiguous results might be very early expression (day 0 or 1) of induced TK or HPRT mutants, marked variations in colony numbers at different expression times or an inverse concentration-related effect. Repeat experiments, paying particular attention to growth conditions, stringent mutant selection, and all the critical culture conditions may be necessary to resolve ambiguous results.

2.5.5 Discussion

Mammalian cell gene mutation assays have a sound genetic and biochemical basis. Defined protocols have been developed for the three most commonly-used cell lines and reproducible results have been produced using a number of chemical mutagens. A limited amount of testing has been done using carcinogens (mainly using the L5178Y TK system) and the role

in predicting carcinogenicity requires further study. Some
systems are capable of determining multiple genetic end-points
(Cole et al., 1982; Gupta & Singh, 1982), and these are
potentially advantageous as mutagen-screening systems.

One of the most important factors influencing the validity
of the data is that the investigator should have a thorough
understanding of the particular cell system in use. This
includes the culture conditions that will support good cell
growth and an awareness of the many possible causes of
sub-optimal growth. Slow growth rate may result in reduced
incorporation of analogues and incomplete kill of wild-type
cells. Other factors that deserve particular emphasis are
described below.

2.5.5.1 Mutant selection

It is very important to ensure stringency of selection for
each particular cell line. Pool sizes differ between cell
lines and under different growth conditions, and the relative
affinity of salvage enzyme for analogue and natural substrate
may differ markedly. The kill curve of the selective agents
used must be carefully checked, and the concentration chosen
should not be within or close to the range in which
exponential fall in survival occurs. This is especially
important if a high and variable spontaneous mutant frequency
is found, as this makes data interpretation particularly
difficult.

2.5.5.2 Expression time

It is essential that a near-optimal expression time for
the induction of mutants should be used if accurate data are
to be obtained for the analysis of concentration-related
effects. The expression time should be carefully defined for
each selective system using a number of mutagens. The use of
a single "standard" expression time may give misleading
results and, ideally, at least two expression times should
always be used so that it is clear that the peak has been
observed. This is particularly important if an unusual
dose-response relationship is obtained, for example few
mutants being induced with increased dose.

2.5.5.3 Cell numbers

Experiments should be designed to maximize the possibility
of statistical analysis of the data. If small effects are to
be detected, it is most important that the spontaneous mutant
frequency should be borne in mind, and that sufficient cells
should be exposed to treatment and cloned in selective medium

to provide reasonable numbers of mutants as a basis for analysis.

2.5.5.4 Metabolic conversion

This is a major area in mammalian cell assays requiring further research. At present, no single experimental design is ideal for detecting all compounds that require metabolic conversion. The factors requiring consideration are species and inducer used for tissue homogenate (S9) preparation, the correct final concentration of the homogenate, and the use of intact cells rather than homogenate. These factors may make a considerable difference to the apparent mutagenicity of the test compound, and the laboratory conducting the test should be able to provide evidence that, using a clearly defined protocol for metabolic conversion, mutagens from different classes of chemicals requiring metabolic activation (e.g., benzo(a)pyrene, N-nitrosodimethylamine, and N-acetyl-2-aminofluorene) induced mutations in a dose-dependent fashion. Flexibility is important as a single compromise protocol may not be appropriate in every case.

2.5.6 Conclusions

Mammalian cell lines have been used in the study of chemically and physically induced specific locus mutations since 1968. Clearly defined methods for mutagenesis assays using cultured mammalian cells have been developed and a detailed examination of the genetic basis of the markers used has been made. Although a number of areas requiring further study remain (Ashby et al., 1985), criteria have been established for an evaluation to be made of the induction of specific locus mutations in mammalian cells, and of the role of such assays in predicting carcinogens.

2.6 The Use of Higher Plants to Detect Mutagenic Chemicals

2.6.1 Introduction

Many of the fundamental concepts of modern genetics were established in higher plants and the term "mutation" was introduced by the Dutch botanist, Hugo de Vries, in 1909, to describe a sudden hereditary change in Oenothera lamarckiana. Plant systems played a major part in early investigations of the genetic changes caused by radiation (Read, 1959; Revell, 1959) and a variety of plants have been used to study the mutagenic effects of chemicals at the gene and chromosome levels. With the increasing concern over the genotoxicity of environmental chemicals for man and the introduction of sophisticated techniques for studying mutations in bacteria, lower plants, insects, and mammalian cells, there has been a loss of interest in the testing of potentially mutagenic chemicals in higher plant systems. This is surprising as plants appear to offer significant advantages over other organisms in certain circumstances, though they have, of course, important limitations.

Techniques for studying mutagenic chemicals have been developed in about 10 species of higher plants and a whole range of specific genetic end-points are available. Mitotic chromosome alterations can be studied in the somatic cells from root tips, or pollen tubes in, for example, barley, the broad bean, or the onion. Pollen mother cells from a number of species are suitable for detecting chemically-induced chromosomal aberrations in meiotic cells. Gene mutations at specific loci can be investigated in maize or soybean plants and multi-locus mutation systems are available in barley and maize. The chromosome systems allow the observation of structural chromosome damage and effects on chromosome segregation and general mitotic function. The chromosomes are morphologically similar, and appear to respond to treatment with mutagens in a similar way to those of mammals and other eukaryotes.

A survey of the literature prepared under the US Environmental Protection Agency Gene-Tox Program (Constantin & Owens, 1982) revealed that about 350 compounds, covering a wide range of chemical classes, had been tested for mutagenic activity in plants. The same authors also compared the results of testing eight model mutagens in plants with the results obtained in other systems. They claimed that the correlation between plant data and results from cultured mammalian cells was at least as good as that with data derived from bacteria and Drosophila. A comparison of the results of testing a series of pesticides in plant root tips and mammalian cells for chromosomal aberrations showed a remarkable qualitative similarity between the two sets of results. However, the data on chromosome damage in mammalian cells for some of the pesticides was not truly representative of the literature on these chemicals. Although a database representing more than 350 compounds tested in plant systems has been assembled, a large proportion of the chemicals tested were shown to be mutagenic in one plant system or another, and there is a significant lack of information on non-mutagenic chemicals.

In spite of the above comments, it is apparent that plant assays possess some advantages over other systems that remain to be fully exploited in the area of genetic toxicology. Chromosome assays on plants are rapid and inexpensive and do not require elaborate laboratory facilities, and a wide range

of genetic end-points is available. However, before the full
potential of plant systems can be exploited, some serious
limitations have to be overcome. There is a lack of knowledge
concerning many of the critical molecular processes in plants,
particularly those influencing the metabolism of foreign
compounds; thus, it is difficult to assess the significance
for mammals, including man, of data derived from plant
experiments. There are also fundamental differences in
structure between plant and mammalian cells. The rigid
cellulose wall of plant cells almost certainly affects the
penetration of certain chemicals and there may be selective
differences between plant and mammalian cells in the kinds of
molecules that can be absorbed. However, the DNA of plants
and animals appears to be similar in structure and function
and the mechanism of protein synthesis seems to be the same.
Higher plants have more cytoplasmic (mitochondrial) DNA than
animal cells and, in addition, the chloroplasts contain DNA.

Mitotic chromosome division in plants follows a similar
course to that in mammalian cells, though meiosis and
gametogenesis are very different. In plants, cell division is
accompanied by the formation of a plate that separates the
daughter cells while in mammals, the cells divide by
constriction of the cytoplasm.

2.6.2   Test systems

Although about 25 different test-systems have been
described in 10 plant species, the following have been
established as practical and useful for testing chemicals for
mutagenic activity:

(a)   mitotic chromosomal damage;
(b)   aberrations in meiotic chromosomes; and
(c)   gene mutations at specific or miltiple loci.

2.6.2.1   Detection of mitotic chromosome damage

Growing root tips of the broad bean, Vicia faba (Ma,
1982b), the onion, Allium cepa (Grant, 1982), the spiderwort,
Tradescantia paludosa (Ma, 1982a), and of barley, Hordeum
vulgare (Constantin & Nilan, 1982) provide a readily available
source of material for studying the damaging effects of
chemicals on chromosomes.

(a)   Vicia faba

The six pairs of chromosomes can be clearly observed at
the metaphase stage of mitosis, and it is possible to identify
all types of chromatid and chromosome aberrations. In

6

addition to conventional metaphase analysis, methods are also available for detecting chromosome damage by counting micronuclei and for recording sister chromatid exchanges. The technique is most suitable for studying water-soluble chemicals, but by using organic solvents, e.g., dimethyl sulfoxide, other compounds can also be tested. Normally, stock solutions of the test compound are added to the growth solution; appropriate buffers should be used to correct extremes of pH. Freshly prepared solution should always be used. The technique (Kihlman, 1971) is relatively simple, and requires only a minimum of laboratory equipment. Seeds are softened by soaking in water for 6 - 12 h, then allowed to germinate in moist vermiculite or similar medium at a temperature of about 19 °C. After germination (4 days), the growing shoot is removed and the seedlings transferred to a tank of water, which should be fully aerated. After 24 h in the tank, primary root growth is sufficiently active for study. It is important to control the pH and temperature of the water as both may affect the frequency of chromosome aberrations induced by a given chemical.

Treatment times may vary between 1 and 24 h, though short treatment times are preferable for the identification of the most sensitive mitotic stages. However, it is conventional to incorporate two or three different treatment times, when testing chemicals of unknown mutagenic activity. The mitotic cycle of Vicia is between 18 and 22 h and, as the interphase stage is the most sensitive to the majority of chemicals, it is necessary to allow a recovery period of about 8 h in the absence of the test chemical. This ensures that roots are fixed and processed at a stage where chromosomes damaged by the chemical will be in the first metaphase after treatment. In some cases, an additional recovery period of 30 - 40 h may be used, so that chromosomes can be examined at the second metaphase. Both treatment and recovery should take place in the dark. Before the roots are fixed, they are transferred to a solution of 0.02 - 0.05% colchicine and agitated in this solution for 2 - 4 h. This treatment blocks the cell cycle at the metaphase stage and leads to an accumulation of metaphase chromosomes that are suitable for analysis.

For most purposes, fixation in ethanol: acetic acid (3:1) gives satisfactory results. This is best carried out at 4 °C (refrigerator temperature) for a minimum of 20 min; fixation from 2 - 24 h is more effective for permanent preparations. For preliminary analysis or when permanent preparations are not required, chromosomes can be stained using the aceto-orcein method. The Feulgen squash technique of Darlington & Lacour (1969) is preferable for permanent slides followed by rapid freezing, dehydration in alcohol, and mounting.

The various kinds of chromosomal aberrations can be scored in metaphase preparations and, for many chemicals, the scoring of chromatid-type aberrations in the first metaphase after treatment gives the most reliable measure of mutagenic activity. However, some compounds, e.g., maleic hydrazide, produce a peak of activity during the second metaphase and this should be determined before a chemical is regarded as inactive. Examination of anaphase chromosomes for fragments and bridges is a useful technique for rapid screening and for obtaining preliminary information on clastogenic (i.e., chromosome-breaking) activity, mitotic delay, and the absence of cell division. Such information is useful for deciding treatment concentrations and times and recovery periods for subsequent metaphase studies. For a detailed description of metaphase and anaphase aberrations, see Kihlman (1971).

Micronuclei resulting from chromosome fragments or lagging chromosomes can be scored at the interphase following treatment (Ma, 1982a), and a technique has been described for investigating sister-chromatid exchanges (SCE) in root tips (Kihlman & Andersson, 1982).

A sufficient number of root tips should be used for each of a wide range of concentrations of the test compound to give an adequate number of data for subsequent interpretation and, if necessary, statistical evaluation. A minimum of 100 metaphase cells should be analysed from at least 10 roots for each experimental group. Doses should be selected within half-log intervals and compounds should be tested up to obviously cytotoxic or inhibitory (i.e., reduction in mitotic index) concentrations. It is usual to conduct preliminary experiments to identify a suitable range of concentrations. More than one exposure period and two or three recovery periods may be necessary to obtain the maximum incidence of chromosome damage and a major objective is to determine a dose-response relationship for chemicals that appear to be mutagenic. Control experiments are needed for each assay and should include a negative control, consisting of roots cultured in the growth solution including any solvent used, and a positive control, consisting of roots treated with a known mutagen such as ethylmethane sulfonate.

Results are usually expressed as the number of aberrations per 100 cells, per group and the number in each experimental group is compared with the values from the negative control group. In most cases, positive results are so obvious that statistical analysis is unnecessary. Where the number of aberrations is low, a simple t-test or Chi-squared test, using a significant level of 1% to determine positive results, is usually adequate.

(b) <u>Allium cepa</u>

Although a number of species of <u>Allium</u> have been used for
genetic studies, the common onion, <u>Allium cepa</u>, has proved to
be the species of choice for root-tip chromosome studies
(Grant, 1982). Mitotic cells of <u>Allium</u> contain 8 pairs of
large chromosomes. The technique for root-tip chromosome
preparations is very similar to that described for <u>Vicia</u>. The
outer scales are removed from young bulbs to expose the root
primordia and they are then supported in a rack over a
suitable tank containing water at 20 °C. Adequate root growth
should be obtained in 2 - 4 days. The roots are then ready
for treatment with the test chemicals followed by processing
and mounting as described above. In an even simpler
technique, <u>Allium cepa</u> seeds are germinated on layers of paper
towelling soaked with the test solution in a culture dish.
Primary roots are usually 0.5 - 1.0 cm long after 3 days, and
they can then be processed for analysis.

(c) <u>Tradescantia paludosa</u>

Compared to <u>Allium</u> and <u>Vicia</u>, only a few chemicals have
been tested for mitotic chromosomal aberrations in
<u>Tradescantia</u>, but it has the advantage that both meiotic and
mitotic chromosomal damage and gene mutations can be tested in
the same species. Dividing cells in the root tip of
<u>Tradescantia</u> contain 12 large metacentric chromosomes. A
large number of roots can be obtained from cuttings from
mature plants in about a week. These rooted cuttings can then
be used for chromosome studies in much the same way as those
of <u>Allium</u> or <u>Vicia</u> (Ahmed & Grant, 1972).

(d) <u>Hordeum vulgare</u>

Both root-tip and shoot-tip cells can be used to
investigate mitotic chromosome changes in barley. The
chromosomes are large, 12 in number, and very suitable for the
rapid scoring of aberrations. The procedure is similar to
that described above. Barley seeds are allowed to germinate
while in contact with the test solution. Five to seven
primary roots develop from each seed and the roots are usually
fixed between 24 and 48 h after germination and then processed
for metaphase chromosome analysis. Squash preparations can be
made from a number of growing points on the developing shoot
and numerous cells are usually available for metaphase
analysis. Frequency of chromosome damage may vary between
root tips and shoot preparations because of differences in the
effectiveness of transport of different chemical molecules
(Constantin & Nilan, 1982).

In general, the root tip procedures are relatively simple and sensitive assays for clastogenic chemicals. The species described have small numbers of large chromosomes, which simplifies analysis, and aberrations can be scored at either metaphase or anaphase. They are more suitable for testing water-soluble compounds than those that are not easily soluble. It should be emphasized that the metabolic pathways required for the activation of many chemicals have not been fully characterized in these plant systems. Thus, the relevance of these results for mammalian cells cannot be properly assessed, at present.

2.6.2.2 Detection of aberrations in meiotic chromosomes

Although the processes of sexual reproduction in plants are greatly different from those in mammals, there are some similarities in meiotic cell division and chromosome behaviour. The induction of anomalies in the chromosomes of, for example, pollen mother cells, may be analagous to meiotic chromosome damage in mammalian reproductive cells, though convincing evidence for this is lacking. A number of plants including Vicia and Hordeum offer relatively easy means of studying meiotic events including numerical (e.g., non-disjunction) as well as structural chromosome changes. A method is also described for counting micronuclei in 4-cell stages as a measure of chromosome breakage (Ma, 1982a). The techniques are simple, involving fixing the flower buds in ethyl alcohol/acetic acid, staining the anthers using a squash technique, and then analysing the chromosomes in the pollen mother cells.

(a) Vicia faba

For the examination of meiotic chromosomes in Vicia, it is necessary to raise the plants to maturity in either growth chambers or glasshouses. This is fairly time-consuming and requires much more space than the root-tip assay. Chemicals can be applied either by spraying in solution on the young flower buds or by exposing the buds to the chemical in the form of a gas or vapour in an appropriate chamber (Tomkins & Grant, 1976). Suitable concentrations of the chemical and exposure times are determined from preliminary experiments and it is usual to allow a recovery period before processing the pollen tubes for the analysis of anaphase cells for bridges and fragments.

(b) Tradescantia paludosa

Strains of T. paludosa that proliferate and propagate easily and quickly under local environmental conditions should be used. A suitable clone should grow to maturity from cuttings in 40 - 60 days. Since the chromosomes of pollen mother cells are not of adequate quality for the detailed analysis of metaphase aberrations, a technique has been developed for detecting chromosome breakage on the basis of micronuclei at the tetrad stage. In practice, the inflorescences are removed from the plant and the stems placed in solutions of the test chemical. Alternatively, the buds can be exposed to gaseous materials in a suitable chamber. The optimum length of treatment is determined experimentally and a recovery period of 24 - 30 h is necessary to allow chromosome damage in early prophase 1 to reach the tetrad stage where micronuclei can be scored. Micronuclei are assumed to be a result of either chromosome fragmentation or of whole chromosomes lost during meiosis and are therefore a measure of both structural damage and aneuploidy (or non-disjunction). It is usual to score between 1000 and 1500 tetrads from each experimental group including both negative and positive controls.

(c) Hordeum vulgare

Chromatid and chromosomal aberrations can be investigated in pollen mother cells (microsporocytes), which are present in large numbers in the developing barley spike. The spike is produced when the shoot apex undergoes a transition from a new leaf promordium to an inflorescence primordium. The spike is collected for cytogenetic analysis at approximately the same time as the last leaf (i.e., the flag leaf) emerges. As meiosis in the pollen mother cells is not synchronized, spikes can be used for testing over a period of up to 40 h during development. Chemicals can be applied by spraying the spike or adjoining areas at selected times, before removing the spikes. The entire spike is fixed in ethanol/acetic acid and processed in the normal way (Constantin & Nilan, 1982).

2.6.2.3 Detection of gene mutations at specific or multiple loci

A specific locus is a region of a chromosome that controls the development of a phenotypic characteristic. It is equivalent to the classical Mendelian gene and can mutate to a new allele with an associated change in phenotype. Although there are a number of specific loci that are potentially useful for studying chemical mutagens, only a few systems are sufficiently well characterized to be used in practice. An example of these is the waxy mutation as expressed in pollen grains of maize.

(a) Waxy locus mutations in Zea mays

Maize has a long history of use in genetic studies and hundreds of genotypically defined strains are available. The pistillate flowers containing the female spores (megaspores) develop on a separate part of the plant to the characteristic tassels containing the male spores (microspores). Tetrads of haploid microspores develop in the anthers through a process of meiosis and then, by mitotic division, the male gametophyte or pollen grain is formed. The haploid, female megaspore develops from the megasporocyte by meiotic division and, after a complex process of mitosis, the female gametophyte is produced.

The waxy locus assay is based on dominance or recessiveness in a gene that determines the presence of amylose in the kernel. In the recessive genotype (wx), the kernels have a waxy appearance and the starch of the endosperm contains only amylopectin. The starch in the dominant (Wx) form consists of a mixture of amylopectin and amylose. Kernels carrying the Wx allele stain a dark blue-black when stained with iodine while wx/wx kernels, which have no amylose, stain a red colour. The waxy phenotype can also be detected in pollen grains using the iodine reaction and this forms the basis of the assay.

The assay can be conducted by the direct treatment of the tassels, which are harvested at an appropriate time and stored in 70% ethanol. Homozygous Wx plants are exposed to the test chemical and forward mutations are detected by a lack of amylose in the iodine-treated pollen. A reverse mutation assay using plants of the Wx/wx genotype can be used in a similar technique.

It is usual to analyse some 250 000 pollen grains per tassel in 5 - 10 plants. The frequency of mutants in pollen from treated plants is compared with that from the untreated controls.

Further details of this and other mutation assays in maize, and information on the application and interpretation of these procedures are given in the review by Plewa (1982).

(b) Chlorophyll-deficient mutations in Hordium vulgare

Chlorophyll synthesis and its control is governed by a large number of genes and a variety of recessive mutations can be detected after treatment of barley seed with mutagens or by exposure of the plant during its complete life cycle. The procedure for detecting chlorophyll-deficient mutations is relatively time-consuming as they are observed in the second (M_2) generation after treatment of the seed. The system is reviewed by Constantin (1976). The waxy pollen test can also be applied in barley (Sulovska et al., 1969).

(c) Somatic mosaicism in Glysine max

The induction of spots of contrasting colour in the leaves of soybean seedlings appears to have many attributes as a useful short-term test for mutagenic chemicals. The spots result from a variety of genetic changes in either meiotic or mitotic cells, the assay can be completed in 4 - 5 weeks, and its requires a minimum of laboratory facilities. The test is based on the Y_{11} locus and its mutation to y_{11}. The homozygous Y_{11} Y_{11} has dark green leaves that may show light green or very dark green spots, the heterozygous Y_{11} y_{11} has light green leaves showing dark green, yellow, or twin (dark green/yellow) spots. Although cytological evidence of the genetic basis of the mosaicism is limited, it has been inferred from the phenotypic expression that the spots may be a result of somatic crossing over, non-disjunction, chromosome deletion, gene mutation, or somatic gene conversion.

In studies on the induction of leaf mosaics, seeds are treated with the test chemical during germination. They are then planted in a non-nutritive medium and grown under controlled conditions in a glasshouse until the second compound leaf unfurls (4 - 5 weeks). The number and type of spots per leaf on each plant is recorded and the numbers of spots on treated plants compared with the untreated control values. An appropriate positive control group (i.e., mitomycin C, N-methyl-N-nitrosourea) is included in each assay. For a detailed review of the assay see Vig (1982).

(d) Somatic gene mutations in Tradescantia

The Tradescantia assay, which involves a change in flower colour from blue to pink, is particularly suitable detecting mutagens in the atmosphere (Schairer et al., 1978). The hybrid clone 4430 is heterozygous for a specific flower colour locus. The dominant blue allele produces the phenotypically blue colour in the petals. The recessive pink phenotype is only expressed by mutation or deletion at the blue allele. The pink colour is detected as pink cells in the stamen or as sectors in the petals. For laboratory studies, cuttings bearing a young inflorescence are treated with liquid or gaseous compounds for periods of a few hours to a number of days. The cuttings are then transferred to growth chambers under standard conditions, until the necessary observations have been carried out. Mutations are expressed as single pink cells or as strings of pink cells in the stamen hairs. Some 40 - 75 hairs can be obtained from each bud. Details of the technique and its application for detecting gaseous mutagens in the environment are given by Van't Hof & Schairer (1982).

2.6.3   Discussion

There are about 10 test systems in plants that can be used to investigate the mutagenic effects of chemicals and they cover a full spectrum of genetic end-points. They range from the rapid and simple root-tip assays for structural chromosome damage to relatively complex tests for specific locus mutations. Plant assays have been used extensively to test chemicals in solution and some of the systems are uniquely fitted for detecting low concentrations of atmospheric mutagens. A test using homosporus ferns (Klewoski, 1978) is being developed for detecting water-borne mutagens in natural waters and effluents.

Although the literature on plant mutagenesis is extensive, there are few data comparing the results observed in plants with those in mammals, and extrapolation between the two remains somewhat tenuous. Some mammalian carcinogens that are known to require metabolic conversion to reactive molecules are detected as mutagens in plant systems (e.g., some nitrosamines). In the limited comparisons available, there is a positive correlation between mutagenicity in plants and mammalian cells. However, there appear to be two serious limitations in the interpretations of the results of plant assays in terms of human hazard. First, though there are data on up to a hundred chemicals in some systems, the majority of the chemicals tested have been mutagens (in some assays as many as 95% of chemicals tested). Thus, many more data on the response of plants to chemicals shown to be non-mutagenic in other systems are required. The second limitation is related to the fundamental differences in the metabolism of foreign compounds between plants and mammals, and information is lacking on the mutagenicity and metabolic mechanisms in plants for many of the major classes of mammalian carcinogens.

In spite of these reservations, it must be recognised that plant systems have many attributes in terms of cost and technical simplicity that recommend their use in specific circumstances for the initial screening of chemicals for mutagenic activity.

2.7 The Drosophila Sex-Linked Recessive Lethal Assay (SLRL)

2.7.1 Introduction

The fruitfly Drosophila melanogaster is a test organism in which it is possible to analyse in vivo heritable mutations and chromosomal aberrations in the same population of treated germ cells. Special strains (stocks) are available or can be constructed to study gonadal or somatic tissue for gene mutations, deletions, and for almost all possible types of chromosomal rearrangements. In addition, special test protocols have been devised to detect aneuploidy resulting from nondisjunctional events. Comparative investigations on the reliability of these different genetic end-points have clearly revealed that the X-linked recessive lethal test is by far the most sensitive and reliable assay in Drosophila to screen compounds for heritable genetic damage. One of the major reasons is that the phenomenon of "recessive lethality" can have different origins: recessive lethals comprise point mutations (intragenic changes), deletions affecting more than one gene, and both small and large rearrangements (Auerbach, 1962a). Thus, a mutagen that only produced gene mutations would not be detected in a test for translocations, but would still be picked up in the recessive lethal assay. In this section, a brief outline of the performance and the most essential points of the recessive lethal method will be given.

2.7.2 Procedure

2.7.2.1 Test organism life cycle

Drosophila melanogaster undergoes complete metamorphosis. The egg produces a larva that undergoes two molts, so that the larval period consists of three stages (instars). The third instar larva becomes a pupa which, in turn, develops into an imago, or adult. Depending on the temperature, this fly requires 9 - 20 days to complete one generation. At 25 °C, the culture temperature preferred in most laboratories, the major stages in the life cycle are: embryonic development, 1 day; first larval instar, 1 day; second larval instar, 1 day; third larval instar, 2 days; prepupa, 4 h; pupa, 4.5 days. Thus, at 25 °C, one generation lasts only 9 - 10 days.

2.7.2.2 Stock cultures

Glass milk bottles of about 200 ml volume are used for stock cultures. For smaller cultures, e.g., pair matings in the recessive lethal test, vials of about 40 ml are used. The culture media most widely used are banana medium and cornmeal medium, i.e., 74.3 g water, 1.5 g agar, 13.5 g molasses, 10.0 g cornmeal, and 0.7 g methyl-p-hydroxybenzoate (to reduce growth of moulds).

2.7.2.3 List of nomenclature

The book of Lindsley & Grell (1968) entitled "Genetic Variations of Drosophila melanogaster" represents the exhaustive compilation of the mutants of Drosophila. This book gives the nomenclature used by Drosophila geneticists, together with a detailed description of mutants, chromosomal aberrations, special balancer chromosomes, cytological markers, and wild-type stocks. This guide is indispensable when working with Drosophila.

2.7.2.4 Equipment and laboratory techniques

There are several detailed descriptions of mutation work on Drosophila, including culture medium, equipment, stock culturing, and handling of flies (Abrahamson & Lewis, 1971; Demerec & Kaufman, 1973; Würgler et al., 1977).

2.7.3   Principle of the recessive lethal assay

Individual chromosomes of Drosophila melanogaster have been labelled X, Y, 2, 3, and 4. The female chromosomes consist of three pairs of autosomes (2, 3, 4) and one pair of rod-shaped X chromosomes. The chromosome complex (2n) of the male has three pairs of autosomes, one X and one J-shaped Y chromosome. The X and Y chromosomes, therefore, are called the sex chromosomes.

The recessive lethal test can be readily designed to detect the induction of heritable genetic lesions in a large part of the Drosophila genome. Two generations are required for the detection of recessive lethals on the X-chromosome, which represents about 20% of the entire genome. It is estimated that about 700 - 800 of the 1000 loci on the X-chromosome can mutate to give rise to recessive lethal mutations.

The most relevant features of the X-chromosomal recessive lethal test (also referred to as sex-linked recessive lethal assay) are illustrated in Fig. 5. Males from a wild-type laboratory strain are treated (or kept untreated as controls) and are then mated (P_1) with virgin females that are homozygous for the X-linked markers B (Bar, semi-dominant; eye restricted to a narrow vertical bar in male and in homozygous female. Heterozygous female has a number of facets intermediate between homozygous female and wild-types) and "w^a" (white-apricot, recessive; eye colour yellowish pink),

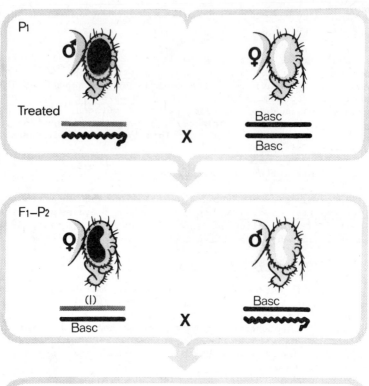

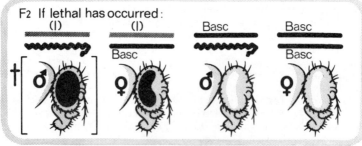

Fig. 5. The Basc test for the detection of X-chromosome recessive lethal mutations.

affecting the shape and colour of the eyes (Lindsley & Grell, 1968). This "Basc" balancer X-chromosome also carries an inversion to prevent crossing-over of a lethal from the treated (paternal) X-chromosome to its homologue in the heterozygotes (F_2-P_2). Thus, the two "marker genes" $\underline{B}$ and "$\underline{w}^a$" serve to distinguish "treated" (paternal) from "untreated" (maternal) chromosomes. The F_1-P_2 generation is intercrossed. In the F_2, which splits into four genotypes that can easily be identified by their different phenotypes, it is possible to distinguish the two classes of flies carrying copies from a treated chromosome (left side) from those that do not (right side). If a complete recessive lethal mutation is induced in an X-bearing germ cell of the treated P_1 male, all the somatic cells of the resulting F_1 female will be heterozygous for this mutation, and also 50% of its eggs will carry it. Half of the F_2 males will be hemizygous carriers for it and will therefore die. But this can be seen only when single-mating is conducted in the F_1, which is an absolute prerequisite for the proper performance of the assay.

Female treatment is not recommended in routine testing procedures, because the females may contain pre-existing lethals that have to be crossed out before starting an experiment. The major advantages of the recessive lethal test are:

(a)   The criterion used to decide whether a mutation is present or not is very objective. The decision is based on whether, in the F_2-generation, one entire class of males is absent or not (Fig. 6). Therefore, personal bias is reduced to a minimum.

(b)   Lethals are much more frequent than other types of genetic lesions, i.e., viable visible mutations or large structural aberrations.

(c)   A representative part of the Drosophila genome is covered by this multi-locus procedure.

2.7.4   Metabolic activation

The organism itself has a complex metabolic system (Vogel et al., 1980). The presence in Drosophila of cytochrome P-450-dependent oxygenase, cytochrome b_5, aryl hydrocarbon hydroxylase, and other components of the xenobiotic-metabolizing enzymes has been demonstrated. There is substantial experimental evidence supporting the conclusion that Drosophila has the enzymic potential for converting a

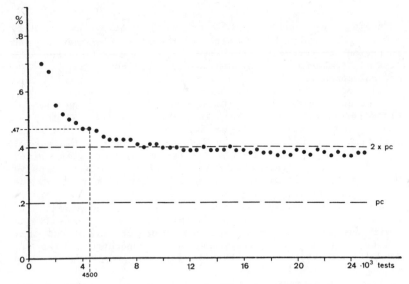

Fig. 6. Lowest mutation frequency significantly different from a control with 10 mutations in 5000 tests (= 0.2%) for increasing numbers of tests in the treated group. From: Würgler et al. (1975).

wide   array   of   pro-mutagens/pro-carcinogens   (about   80 pro-carcinogens to date) into genetically-active species.

2.7.5   Test performance

2.7.5.1   Treatment procedures

Chemicals are most commonly administered to Drosophila, either by injection into the body cavity or by feeding, at the adult or larval stage. Other methods of treating flies include treatment through inhalation or using aerosols. Adult males are recommended for testing purposes, since females are more readily sterilized by chemicals and have, so far, proved more refractory to the induction of heritable genetic changes.

Experience with several classes and types of mutagens indicates the importance of a flexible protocol, when using the recessive lethal assay. There are several examples in which the route of administration has been shown to have a profound effect on the mutagenicity detected. Injection seems to be more reliable for the detection of highly reactive mutagens   such   as   the   unstable   beta-propionylactone   and chloroethylene oxide. Adult feeding is more effective in cases where a single injection (pulse treatment) is highly toxic,   as   has   been   demonstrated   with   the   carcinogen N-nitrosodiethylamide (DEN). Several solvents (ethanol, Tween

60, Tween 80, special fat emulsions) can be used to dissolve
or emulsify chemicals of low water solubility. The use of
DMSO and DMF should be avoided. These solvents have recently
been shown to inhibit chemical mutagenesis in some
pro-carcinogens by blocking their metabolic activation
(Zijlstra et al., 1984).

2.7.5.2 Toxicity tests

Pilot studies should give concentration-mortality
relationships to express the general biological reactivity of
the chemical under test. The availability of such toxicity
data aids the adequate design of the genetic studies and, if
the compound under test is a mutagen, provides the condition
that will produce the maximum yield of mutations without
killing the animal as a result of lethal overdose. Thus,
pilot studies should give an approximate idea of the possible
toxicity (LD_{50}) of the test compound. Technical aspects of
toxicity tests are described by Würgler et al. (1977). Actual
results of toxicity tests with a series of monofunctional
alkylating agents were reported by Vogel & Natarajan (1979).
Regarding the general testing strategy, the highest possible
concentrations that can be used for testing for recessive
lethal mutations should be used first. Acute toxicity,
reduced fertility, and solubility problems may then be the
limiting factors. Use of two different dose levels is
recommended, i.e., the MTD (maximum tolerated dose) and 1/4 or
1/5 of it.

2.7.5.3 Brooding

It is well known that chemical mutagens often exhibit
stage specificity, i.e., show more or less pronounced
mutagenic effects at different stages in germ-cell
development. It is, therefore, essential to analyse the
progeny from treated spermatozoa, late and early spermatids,
and spermatocytes. Analysis of offspring from treated
spermatid stages is of particular importance because there is
considerable evidence, derived from experiments with
alkaryltriazenes, nitrosamines, and other pro-mutagens, that
release of ultimate mutagenic metabolites from the parent
pro-mutagen takes place directly in metabolically-active
spermatid stages, whereas spermatocytes are highly susceptible
to killing. On the other hand, there seems no need to include
in the test the analysis of spermatogonia, because there are
only few cases of mutagens that affect spermatogonia, but are
not active in meiotic or postmeiotic cells (Auerbach, 1962b).
With the brooding technique, the spatial pattern of
spermatogenesis is translated into a temporal pattern of

successive broods. Treated wild-type males are therefore re-mated at regular intervals of 2 - 3 days with fresh virgin Basc females. An excess of 3 - 5 females per male serves to sample all germ cells that are in the mature stage. A total sampling period of 7 - 9 days (3 to 4 broods) is considered sufficient for mutagen testing.

2.7.5.4 Control and replicate experiments: sample size

Würgler et al. (1975) prepared sample-size tables that are very helpful for adequately planning recessive lethal tests. The most significant points in this respect are:

(a) the dependence of the outcome of the genetic test on the number of chromosomes tested;

(b) the dependence of the result on the frequency of spontaneous mutations; and

(c) on statistical grounds, the optimal number of tests to be performed.

It is essential that, before starting a study, particular attention should be paid to these statistical questions. To give an example, with a spontaneous mutation frequency of 0.2% lethals (10 lethals in 5000 progeny) and a sample size of 4500 in the treated group, 0.47% was the lowest value to prove statistically that a mutagenic effect was observed (Fig. 6). It is also obvious from Fig. 6 that an increase in the number of tested chromosomes above 5000 does not really help to improve the resolving power of the assay. The most effective way of planning a study in order to achieve results of statistical significance is to test about equal numbers of chromosomes in the control and the treated groups.

Two studies, consisting of three successive broods each, can be carried out easily within one week, with the aid of one technician. If 600 - 800 cultures are set up for each brood, there is a testing capacity of 1800 - 2400 chromosomes per study. One to two replicate studies should be sufficient to classify a given test substance. Complicated cases with mutation frequencies slightly higher than the spontaneous background, will need further studies. On the average, 80 man-hours are involved in testing an unknown compound.

Experience with several tester stocks has shown that the spontaneous mutability (about 0.1 - 0.2%) remains fairly constant over the years. Initially, control studies should be run concurrently; after more experience, concurrent control studies are not mandatory, if the recessive lethal test is either clearly positive (> 1 - 2% lethals) or negative

(lethal frequency $\leq$ historical controls from the same
laboratory). If the percentage of lethals falls between the
historical control and 1%, concurrent control runs are
obligatory. At least one replicate study should be conducted
in all cases.

2.7.5.5 Literature

Performance of, and possible pitfalls in, the recessive
lethal test have been extensively described by Auerbach
(1962a), Abrahamson & Lewis (1971), and Würgler et al. (1977).

2.7.6 Data processing and presentation

The experimental data to be reported should include the
strains and mating schedule used, the number of chromosomes
tested, and both the number and percentage of lethals. The
aim of a study is to find out whether the mutation frequency
obtained from the treated group is significantly higher than
the spontaneous background. After subtracting from the total
number of F_2 cultures those that are sterile, the
experimental data consist of the following numerical values:

Nc = number of tested X-chromosomes (number of progeny) in
the control group;

Mc = number of recessive lethals in the control group;

Nt = number of tested X-chromosomes (number of progeny) in
the treated group; and

Mt = number of recessive lethals found in the treated
group.

The basic question to be answered is: is the mutation
frequency pt (%) = Mt/Nt x 100, determined for the treated
group, significantly higher than pc = Mc/Nc x 100 for the
control? For statistical consideration of the data, the
simple significance test developed by Kastenbaum & Bowman
(1970) should be applied. Statistical analysis of
mutagenicity data from the recessive lethal assay is further
described by Würgler et al. (1975, 1977).

2.7.7 Discussion

2.7.7.1 Disadvantages of the recessive lethal test

The scoring of induced recessive lethal mutations is a
highly objective method of exploring the mutagenic potential

of a chemical. Nevertheless, there are a few cases of misclassification through incorrect performance of the test. It may, therefore, be profitable to summarize some of the obvious problems that can arise in the design of such studies:

(a)   As a standard rule, single-mating (one male and 3 - 5 females) should be applied to identify the very rare cases of spontaneous clusters, i.e., mutants of common origin. It is then possible to keep track of the F_1 family of cultures derived from each P_1 culture. Clusters will tend to appear in families. If, in postmeiotic broods, large clusters of lethals are observed among F_2 progeny derived from the same P_1 male, it is recommended that these should be eliminated from the final score, because they may reflect spontaneous mutations that arose in dividing spermatogonia during the development of that particular P_1 male.

(b)   Great care must be exercised in the scheme to ensure the use of virgin females in the P-generation. Thus, all F_1 females must be heterozygous for the treated X-chromosome and the Basc balancer chromosome, and at least three of the four different phenotypes must be present in the F_2 generation.

2.7.7.2 Weak mutagens and non-mutagens

Relatively large sample sizes are needed to discriminate between weak mutagens and non-mutagens. It is possible to use either concurrent negative controls, or historical controls. In the latter case, at least 10 000 control tests (chromosomes) should exist for a particular tester strain and each particular solvent (e.g., Tween 80/ethanol). Gocke et al. (1982) reported a very extensive set of historical controls, collected over many years. It has to be stressed that results obtained with a large number of tests, but with only one type of exposure or application, are only informative with regard to that particular set of experimental conditions. Recent instances of weak mutagenic activity in the recessive lethal test are provided in an extensive study on some carcinogenic polycyclic hydrocarbons and aromatic amines (Vogel et al., 1983). No single technique (injection; feeding) was found to be suitable for all the carcinogens investigated; hence, very extensive experiments had to be carried out, using a flexible test protocol.

2.7.7.3 Data base

The recessive lethal assay has been well developed and calibrated against a wide array of direct-acting agents and pro-mutagens. Interlaboratory variability has not been a problem with this assay. According to a report of the US EPA Gene-Tox Program, 421 compounds have been tested in the recessive lethal assay (Lee et al., 1983). Of these, 198 compounds were found to be positive and 46 negative, at the highest concentration tested. A third group containing as many as 177 compounds, was not classified as either positive or negative, because the very rigid criterion used was the test of at least 7000 chromosomes in both the control and the treated groups (per dose level), with a spontaneous frequency of 0.2%. With the fulfillment of this criterion, it would it would be possible to detect a doubling of the recessive lethal frequency (Lee et al., 1983). The problem with this approach is that flexibility is diminished, and that too much weight is put on one experimental condition. The alternative procedure, which seems more realistic in view of the fact that Drosophila constitutes a very complex metabolic system, would be to use a flexible test protocol in studies with weak mutagens. Reliance should not be placed on a large number of chromosomes tested at only one concentration. A variety of experimental conditions (e.g., injections versus feeding) can be used to identify optimal experimental conditions for a given genotoxic agent. A good example of the latter approach is the demonstration by Zijlstra & Vogel (1984) that 7,12-dimethyl-benz(a)anthracene, methyltosylate, and nor-nitrogen mustard are strongly mutagenic, weakly mutagenic, or even ineffective in the recessive lethal assay, depending on the route of administration used.

2.7.7.4 Correlation with mammalian carcinogenicity data

In the Gene-Tox report by Lee et al. (1983), there were 62 compounds that could be classified as positive or negative for both carcinogenesis in mammals and mutagenesis in the recessive lethal assay. Of the 62 compounds, there was agreement between carcinogenic activity and mutagenesis classification in 56 cases (50 positive and 6 negative), i.e., 90% would have been correctly classified as to carcinogenicity using only the SLRL test. The data were derived from a list in which 198 National Cancer Institute (NCI) bioassays were evaluated for carcinogenicity (Griesemer & Cueto, 1980).

In another comparative analysis (Vogel et al., 1980), 85 out of 107 carcinogens (79%) were found to be mutagenic in Drosophila. Of the remaining compounds, 17 were negative and another 5 were not sufficiently tested to reach meaningful conclusions. The documentation by Vogel et al. (1980) is based predominantly on the 142 chemicals considered in the IARC Monographs volumes 1 – 20 for which there is "sufficient evidence of carcinogenicity" in experimental animals, according to evaluations by expert committees (IARC, 1979). A second source for the documentation of carcinogenicity data was a list prepared by the US EPA (1976).

2.7.7.5 Recent developments

The recessive lethal assay is a relatively time-consuming method compared with systems using bacteria or lower eukaryotes. This disadvantage may, however, be offset in the future when, in addition to overall metabolic considerations, attention is directed to differences in metabolism existing between somatic and gonadal tissue, as was recently demonstrated for the inducibility of AHH (aryl hydrocarbon hydroxylase) activity. Thus, somatic assay systems might be particularly valuable as a complement to recessive lethal tests on the germ line. One system is based on eye-colour markers (Becker, 1966), and another on wing-hair markers (Garcia-Bellido et al., 1976). Both systems are currently under validation in several laboratories (Graf et al., 1983; Vogel et al., 1983). With the white/white-coral system (Becker, 1966), which has been calibrated against 35 reference mutagens, it is possible to test about 4 – 6 chemicals in 2 weeks. Moreover, tests based on the detection of genetic changes in somatic cells have the advantage that they can be performed within one generation.

2.8 In Vivo Cytogenetics: Bone Marrow Metaphase Analysis and Micronucleus Test

2.8.1 Introduction

In vivo bone marrow tests, which include metaphase chromosome analysis, and the micronucleus assay are used to identify clastogenic compounds, that is, those that are capable of inducing structural changes in chromosomes. Chromosomal aberrations are analysed in mitotic metaphases from proliferating tissue, such as bone marrow samples from laboratory animals. In the micronucleus test, clastogenic effects can be measured indirectly by counting small nuclei in interphase cells formed from acentric chromosome fragments or whole chromosomes.

Both tests are widely used, and they are regarded as of particular importance by many regulatory authorities, because, in the whole animal, the obvious deficiencies in artificial metabolic activation systems used in <u>in vitro</u> systems are avoided.

2.8.1.1 Current understanding of the formation of chromosomal aberrations

Chromosomal aberrations occur because of lesions in the DNA that lead to discontinuities in the DNA double helix. The primary lesions, which include single- and double-strand breaks, base damage, DNA-DNA and DNA-protein crosslinks, alkylations at base or phosphate groups, intercalations, thymine dimers, apurinic and apyrimidinic sites, are recognized by DNA-repair processes. Therefore, the lesions may be corrected or transformed, to restitute the original base sequence or produce chromosomal aberrations and/or gene mutations.

The breakage-reunion hypothesis (Sax, 1938) implies that a discontinuity in the DNA may be stabilized to appear as a break at metaphase. Alternatively, the discontinuity may be restituted by repair processes to the original state, whereby the chromosome does not exhibit visible structural changes. Two DNA discontinuities in temporal and spatial proximity may interact in the reunion of the broken ends, thus forming exchange configurations. The exchange hypothesis (Revell, 1959) postulates that all aberrations are the result of exchange processes that involve interaction between two local instabilities in close proximity. Experimental data have been provided in support of both hypotheses.

Recent experimental results support the breakage-first hypothesis. The evidence for double-strand breaks being the ultimate DNA lesion for chromosomal aberrations has been summarized by Obe et al. (1982). Double-strand breaks lead directly to chromosomal aberrations; all other primary lesions require transformation to double-strand breaks by DNA replication and/or repair processes.

Double-strand breaks can be induced directly by ionizing radiation and S-independent chemicals, e.g., bleomycin. Double-strand breaks may lead to an immediate fixation of the aberration by misrepair. Depending on the time of induction within the cell cycle, the types of aberrations observed at the succeeding metaphase are of a chromosome (from G_1) or chromatid (from G_2) nature, i.e., involve both or only one chromatid (Evans, 1962). Most chemical mutagens do not cause double-strand breaks directly. The preliminary lesions are transformed in S-phase, and the aberrations observed at metaphase are of the chromatid type (Evans & Scott, 1964). A classification of chemicals according to their mode of action during the different phases of the cell cycle was given by Bender et al. (1974) and is still valid (Brewen & Stetka, 1982).

2.8.1.2 Classification of chromosomal aberrations

Aberrations are divided into chromatid-type and chromosome-type, the first involving only one chromatid, the latter, both chromatids at identical sites. Furthermore, breaks can be distinguished from exchange configurations by their physical appearance at metaphase rather than by their mode of formation. Breaks are true discontinuities with clearly dislocated fragments and also include fragments without obvious origin. They should not be confused with achromatic lesions (gaps), which do not represent true discontinuity in the DNA. It is generally assumed that gaps are sites of despiralization in the metaphase chromosome that render the DNA non-visible under light microscopy. It has been proposed that an achromatic lesion may actually be a single-strand break in the DNA double helix as a result of incomplete excision repair and, thus, may represent a point of possible instability (Bender et al., 1974). Therefore, gaps are always noted but reported separately from true chromosomal aberrations.

Exchange configurations can be subdivided into intrachanges, i.e., exchange within one chromosome, and interchanges, i.e., exchange between two chromosomes. The classification into intra- and interchanges applies to chromatid- as well as to chromosome-type aberrations. Depending on the location of the original discontinuities and the ways of reunion, further classification of exchanges is possible such as symmetrical or asymmetrical, complete or incomplete. The terminology is complex but has been clearly reviewed by Savage (1976) and Scott et al. (1983).

The majority of aberrations observed at first metaphase after exposure are lethal to the cell that carries them or to the daughter cells. Whenever acentric fragments are formed, genetic imbalance will result. In the case of chromosome-type aberrations, both daughter cells will die, since both chromatids are affected. In some cases of chromatid-type aberrations, only one chromatid is affected and only one of the daughter cells may die. Only symmetrical forms of chromosome or chromatid exchanges, with no loss of genetic material, will survive cell division and be transmitted to future cell generations. Chromatid-type aberrations that survive the first division are converted to derived chromosome-type aberrations. The balanced "stable" types of aberrations are reciprocal translocations and inversions. Since there is no rule without exceptions, the occasional balance of genetic material will allow cell survival. Chromosomal syndromes in human diseases such as Cri du Chat (deletion of chromosome 5) or Down's syndrome (trisomy 21) are

due to structural or numerical chromosomes changes, i.e.,
genetic imbalance.

Some more unspecific chromosomal changes should be
mentioned for the sake of completeness. So-called
sub-chromatid aberrations have been primarily observed at
anaphase, most typically as "side arm bridges", after exposure
of cells to ionizing radiation during prophase of cell
division. A model of sub-chromatid aberrations has been
discussed by Klasterska et al. (1976). However, another
phenomenon, namely chromosome stickiness, cannot be
discriminated from subchromatid aberrations, when cells are
scored at metaphase rather than anaphase.

Chromosome shattering can be seen at metaphase, similarly
chromosome pulverisation has been described. There is no
clear distinction between these two phenomena, which simply
represent different degrees of damage inflicted on the
chromosomes. In the case of shattering, chromosomes appear to
have been broken up into many small pieces of various
lengths. Sometimes just a few, sometimes all, chromosomes are
shattered but usually intact chromosomes or conventional
chromatid-type aberrations remain recognizable. In cells with
pulverisation, the chromosomes can be reduced to masses of
fragments. The phenomenon of premature chromosome
condensation (PCC) is sometimes confused with shattering or
pulverisation. However, its appearance is quite different.
Thin chromosomal fragments of various lengths lie among the
debris. The PCC phenomenon was shown to arise from the
virus-mediated fusion of a cell in division to a cell in
S-phase, which brings about visualization (condensation) of
chromosomes in the process of duplication (Johnson & Rao,
1970). PCC was also described in Chinese hamster bone marrow
after chemical treatment (Kürten & Obe, 1975). Here, it was
explained as condensation of chromatin in micronuclei, induced
by mitotic condensation of the chromosomes in the main nuclei
while the micronuclei were still in S-phase.

Polyploidy and endoreduplication are frequently described
in cultured cells, though they are less often seen in
bone-marrow material. Although it is important to assess
aneuploidy, the routine scoring of numerical aberrations in
bone-marrow metaphases is not recommended, because deviations
in chromosome number often arise as preparational artifacts.

2.8.1.3 The basis for micronucleus formation

Micronuclei originate from chromosomal material that has
lagged in anaphase. In the course of mitosis, this material
is distributed to only one of the daughter cells. It may be
included in the main nucleus or form one or more separate
small nuclei, i.e., micronuclei. The micronuclei mainly

consist of acentric fragments as demonstrated by DNA content measurements (Heddle & Carrano, 1977). They may also consist of entire chromosomes and may result from non-disjunction due to malfunction of the spindle apparatus. These larger micronuclei are formed by spindle poisons (Yamamoto & Kikuchi, 1980). Micronuclei can be observed in any cell type of proliferating tissue. They are, however, most easily recognized in cells without the main nucleus, namely erythrocytes.

The scoring of micronuclei in bone-marrow cells was proposed as a screening-test by Boller & Schmid (1970) and Heddle (1973). The frequency of micronuclei can be evaluated most readily in young erythrocytes, shortly after the main nucleus is expelled. The young ones are termed polychromatic erythrocytes (PCEs), the mature ones normochromatic erythrocytes (NCEs). With conventional staining techniques, PCEs stain bluish to purple because of the high content of ribonucleic acid in the cytoplasm. NCEs stain reddish to yellow. The PCEs are also slightly larger than the NCEs.

In mouse-bone marrow, the maturing erythroblasts go through six or seven cell divisions with a cell-cycle length of about 10 h (Cole et al., 1979). About 10 h after the last mitotic division, the expulsion of the main nucleus is completed and the resulting PCE remains in the bone marrow for another 10 h. Treatment-induced micronuclei derived from chromosomal fragments produced during the preceeding cell cycle will thus appear in PCEs not earlier than 10 h after injection of the animal with the test chemical. Experience with known chemical mutagens has shown that, in fact, micronuclei appear much later than this. Jenssen & Ramel (1978) demonstrated by simultaneous treatment of mice with methyl methanesulfonate (MMS) and ^{3}H-thymidine labelling that nuclear expulsion was delayed by about 9 h. Even though an increase in micronuclei levels compared with controls was already seen after 12 h, the curve rose steeply between 18 and 24 h, corresponding to the MMC-induced delay of the last cell cycle up to nuclear expulsion.

2.8.2   Procedure

Detailed experimental procedures are described by Adler (1985).

2.8.2.1   Experimental animals

Bone-marrow studies can be carried out with most laboratory mammals. Chinese hamsters may be preferred for metaphase analysis because of their low chromosome number (2n = 22) and their readily-distinguishable chromosomes. Mice

(2n = 40) or rats (2n = 42) are also frequently used. For the micronucleus test, the use of rats is less convenient. Rat tissue is rich in mast cells. In the course of bone marrow preparation, these cells shed granules containing heparin, which stain in a similar manner to micronuclei, and thus, make scoring of true micronuclei rather difficult.

The animals used in bone-marrow studies should be young adults. The high proliferative activity and the low fat content of bone marrow in young animals favour the quality of the preparations. Each group of test animals should consist of equal numbers of males and females to allow for sex differences in response to the treatment.

2.8.2.2 Treatment and sampling

The treatment should generally comprise a single application of the test compound, followed by multiple sampling of groups of animals at different times (Preston et al., 1981). The most commonly used routes of application are intraperitoneal injection and oral intubation. Other routes of application, e.g., inhalation, are possible. The time of maximum response may vary from chemical to chemical, depending on the sensitive cell-cycle stage and the influence of the chemical on cell-cycle length. Moreover, absorption, distribution, and metabolism may influence the optimum interval between treatment and sampling. Therefore, a single, generally applicable sampling time cannot be recommended. The central sampling interval after dosing is usually 24 h for chromosome analysis and 30 h for the micronucleus test. In addition, one earlier and one later sampling interval should be used, e.g., between 12 - 18 and 36 - 48 h for metaphase analysis and 12 - 18 and 60 - 72 h for the micronucleus test.

Earlier publications on bone-marrow cytogenetics and the micronucleus test (Matter & Schmid, 1971; Schmid et al., 1971) recommended two treatments with a 24-h interval between the two. Other authors have used 5 daily applications of the test compound. The single treatment schedule is preferable for the following reasons:

(a) Cell killing

Chromosomal aberrations do not accumulate over successive cell-cycles, because, in most cases, they are cell-lethal. Thus, true clastogens also kill cells. In repeated treatment schedules, the first dose kills off the most sensitive cells leaving a changed cell population of more resistant cells for the following treatments.

(b) <u>Analysis of first post-treatment mitosis</u>

Chromosomal aberrations can only be assessed quantitatively if scored at the first post-treatment mitosis. If multiple treatments are applied at 24-h intervals, the cells damaged by the first application will have gone through one or more cell divisions. Aberrations that are cell-lethal will have been lost by death of the cells. Scorable chromatid-type aberrations, if the cells have not been rendered non-viable, will have transformed into derived chromosome-type aberrations. These can only be recognized with banding techniques and karyotyping of each cell, a procedure that is too laborious for screening purposes. Thus, the chromatid-type aberrations scored after long-term treatments will represent only the effect of treatment on the penultimate cell cycle.

In theory, micronuclei may accumulate after treatment of two or more cell cycles, since they are scored in a cell type that does not undergo further cell division (Salamone et al., 1980). However, as with metaphase analysis, the cell-killing effect will adversely influence the micronucleus yields after repetitive treatment of the proliferating precursor cells. In order to measure the accumulation of damage under conditions of low cell-toxicity, the spacing of treatment should be governed by the length of the cell-cycle. Cole et al. (1981) recommend that for studies using the bone marrow of adult mice, 10-h intervals should be used and erythrocytes should be sampled 25 h after the last treatment. But, even if cell killing does not occur at low doses, cell-cycle delay caused by the test chemical, as described in the previous section for MMS, may defeat the purpose of the study.

Repeated treatment schedules can occasionally be justified for pharmacological reasons. For example, if a compound requires metabolic activation by an enzyme that is induced by the chemical itself, it can be argued that, to establish the necessary enzyme level, the compound should be administered several times. However, 7,12-dimenthylbenz(a)anthrazene and benzo(a)pyrene, which are metabolized by self-induced enzyme systems, readily induced micronuclei after a single application and required relatively late sampling (36 h or 48/72 h) (Salamone et al., 1980; Kliesch et al., 1982). An increase in micronuclei was not observed after benzo(a)pyrene was adminstered in a 5-day treatment schedule (Bruce & Heddle, 1979). Thus, for the micronucleus test, the advantage of repeated treatments is questionable.

Because of cell-killing effects and the necessity to analyse first post-treatment mitoses, long-term treatments are not suitable for chromosome studies with proliferating tissues. If, for whatever reason, prolonged treatment is required, e.g., in a feeding study, non-proliferating cells such as peripheral lymphocytes should be sampled from the treated animals. These cells can be stimulated to cycle in vitro so that it is possible to score first mitoses after treatment or to count micronuclei in second interphase cells.

2.8.2.3 Dose levels

The choice of test dose levels is based on the maximum tolerated dose (MTD) of the compound in the species used for the test. The MTD is defined by the cellularity of the bone marrow and the yield of analysable metaphases or PCEs. A rule of thumb is to use the MTD as the highest dose. To accept a positive result, it is usually necessary to demonstrate an increase in effect with increasing dose. If the test results are negative, the conclusion is only acceptable when two or three dose levels have been tested or the test has been repeated. Testing with additional dose levels can be restricted to the interval of maximum effect with the highest dose level or to the central sampling interval in case of negative results with the highest dose, bearing in mind the fact that cell-cycle delay is related, not only to the nature of the chemical, but also to the dose level.

2.8.2.4 Number of cells scored per animal

The number of metaphases scored or PCEs counted per animal is governed by the number of animals in each group and the statistical procedure used for planning and evaluating the study. At least 500 metaphases or 4000 PCEs should be scored for a single-dose group.

2.8.2.5 Positive and negative controls

A negative vehicle-control (solvent) is an essential part of each study. A positive control is generally required. The positive control is only meaningful if it demonstrates the test sensitivity with the lowest positive dose of a known clastogen, e.g., 0.16 mg/kg of mitomycin C or 3.1 mg/kg of procarbazine (Kliesch et al., 1982). When the chemical under test is given in repeated treatments, the positive control has to demonstrate that treatment with a known clastogen at low dose levels produces an effect.

2.8.2.6 Preparation procedure for bone-marrow metaphases

The preparation procedure has been described in detail by Dean (1969). Animals are injected with colchicine or Colcemid solutions prior to bone marrow sampling, in order to accumulate metaphases. Other spindle poisons can also be used. Dose levels and timing depend on the animal species. For mice, 4 mg colchicine/kg body weight is usually given, 1 - 1.5 h prior to sacrifice. Chinese hamsters require a longer period of colchicine treatment. In vitro colchicine treatment is also possible, after collection of bone marrow (Tjio & Wang, 1965).

Bone marrow is flushed from the femur into a neutral medium such as 2.2% sodium citrate, Hank's balanced salt solution (HBSS). After the sampling of bone marrow from all animals into individual centrifuge tubes is completed, the cells are centrifuged for 5 min at 100 x 6. The supernatant is discarded completely and a hypotonic solution is slowly added while agitating the tube to disperse the pellet. The hypotonic medium can be 1% sodium citrate, 0.56% potassium chloride, or the medium diluted with distilled water (1:1). The duration of the hypotonic treatment depends on the animal species and ranges from 15 to 30 min at room temperature. Hypotonic effects may be intensified at 37 °C; however, clumping of cells due to collagens and fat in the bone marrow is also increased. After centrifugation, at the end of hypotonic treatment, the cells are fixed by the addition drop-wise of freshly prepared cold methanol/acetic acid mixture (3:1) to the resuspended pellet. The fixative is changed 3 times. In between, the cell suspensions should be stored in the refrigerator and can remain there overnight before slide making. It is essential that fresh fixative be prepared just prior to fixation; it cannot be kept overnight because ester formation will weaken the fixation effect.

For slide making, the most crucial factor is that the glass slides are absolutely clean and grease-free. They can be kept in 70% alcohol (overnight), used wet, and then flame-dried which facilitates chromosome spreading. Other methods of slide making include cooling the slides in an ice-box before use or storing them in cold distilled water and using them wet. Shortly after the cell suspension has been applied (2 - 3 drops per slide), they can be dried on a warm plate.

Slides are usually stained for 10 min in a 5% Giemsa solution (pH 6.8). The staining solutions have to be filtered, immediately before use. The stained slides are washed in distilled water, air-dried, cleared in xylene, and cover-slipped using a suitable mounting medium. Staining with 2% acetic orcein for 30 min is also suitable.

2.8.2.7 Preparation procedure for micronuclei

The method, which has been described in detail by Matter & Schmid (1971), Heddle (1973), and Schmid (1976), includes the following basic steps. Bone marrow is flushed from the femur into fetal calf serum, the cells are centrifuged for 5 min at 100 x g, and the supernatant is discarded as completely as possible. The pellet is resuspended and care should be taken to prevent the loss of any material into the wide part of the pasteur pipette. One drop of the bone-marrow suspension is placed on one end of a clean, grease-free slide, and pulled behind a glass cover slip to produce a cone of bone-marrow smear. The slides are air-dried before staining, possibly overnight, and double-stained with May-Grünwald and Giemsa as described by Schmid (1976). The only change adapted by various laboratories is the replacement of distilled water by phosphate buffer (pH 6.8) for the Giemsa solution.

2.8.2.8 Microscopic analysis

Slides are coded before scoring and only decoded after scoring of the entire study is completed.

(a) Chromosomal aberrations at metaphase

Slides are screened for analysable metaphases under low-power magnification (16 or 25 x objective). High magnification (oil immersion objective) is used for examination of each individual metaphase. Only cells with the complete number of centromeres are included. Each aberration is noted separately on a scoring sheet. Vernier readings can be taken for all cells or only for those that carry an aberration.

Selection of analysable metaphases may pose a certain bias. Criteria for rejecting a metaphase include: incomplete number of centromeres; loss of chromatid alignement and/or centromere splitting due to extended colchicine treatment; extensive overlap of chromosomes; and poor fixation of the chromosomes.

The mitotic index, which is the fraction of cells in a given population that undergo mitosis at a given time, indicates cell proliferation activity. The number of mitoses should be determined for each animal by counting 500 nuclei. Changes in the mitotic index reflect the cytotoxic effect of the treatment.

(b) Micronuclei in polychromatic erythrocytes (PCEs)

Polychromatic erythrocytes are counted in each field of high-power magnification (oil immersion objective), and the number of those with micronuclei is determined. The ratio of PCEs to NCEs is established for each animal by counting a total of 1000 erythrocytes. Changes in the ratio of PCEs to

NCEs reflect the cytotoxic effect of the treatment. The number of NCEs with micronuclei is also noted.

2.8.3 Data processing and presentation

2.8.3.1 Chromosomal aberrations

From the raw data on the scoring sheets, two ways of tabulating the individual animal data should be used, i.e., number of aberrations per cell, and number of cells with aberrations. These express the severity of damage to the affected cell, and to the cell population, respectively. In the individual animal data sheets, results from each animal within one experimental group are listed, and the various types of aberrations are recorded. In the summary reporting sheets, mean values and standard deviations over all animals are given for the various experimental groups. While gaps and breaks are kept separate in the summary reports, the various forms of exchange can be summarized, but should be separated according to chromatid- or chromosome-type. Two columns should give the mean of all aberrations per cell (including and excluding gaps) and the average percent of cells with aberrations (including and excluding gaps). Changes in the mitotic index should be reported separately.

2.8.3.2 Micronuclei

Individual animal-report sheets are compiled from the raw data. They contain the total number of PCEs counted, the ratio of PCEs to NCEs, and the number of PCEs with micronuclei. From the individual animal reporting sheets, the summary report is compiled by giving the average frequency of micronucleated PCEs (for each experimental group), the average ratio of PCEs/NCEs, and the average micronucleated NCEs.

2.8.3.3 Statistical evaluation

Katz (1978) stresses the point that the best designed studies are those with approximately equal numbers of individuals in the experimental and control groups. He also points out that the minimum number of animals in the study is governed by the spontaneous incidence and the required sensitivity.

A statistical design for the micronucleus test was described by Mackey & MacGregor (1979). They used a sequential sampling strategy and based the statistical analysis on the negative binomial distribution or the binomial distribution. The number of animals in their design was not fixed and the number of PCEs per animal was arbitrarily chosen to be either 500 or 1000. Decision limits were given on the basis of the spontaneous micronucleus incidence of 2/1000, a required 3-fold increase for a positive result and an 0.01 probability of error to both sides. Sampling and treatment of animals in this design have to be continued as long as the cumulative micronucleus counts fall between the given limits.

Equally as important as the number of animals, is the number of cells scored. This again depends on the spontaneous frequency of the parameter under test and the required increase for a positive result. Grafe & Vollmar (1977) published a table that related these two factors to the minimum number of cells required in the micronucleus test. The table was based on the assumption of binomial distribution and a probability of error of 0.05. According to the table, a sample of 15 700 cells would be necessary to recognize an increase by a factor of 2 over the spontaneous micronucleus frequency of 2/1000. This approach is useful when the total number of cells is scored with no regard for interanimal variation. However, because there is usually a lack of homogeneity between treated animals, it is the number of animals in the experimental group that determines the precision of the statistical procedure rather than the total number of cells scored.

The inadequacy of the currently available statistical approaches lies in the fact that the number of cells per animal or the number of animals per group is chosen arbitrarily. So far, none of the published recommendations for the statistical planning and evaluation of cytogenetic in vivo tests (including the micronucleus test) has dealt with the problem of interanimal and within-animal variability in treated groups. The distribution of cytogenetic variables remains debatable and difficult to determine.

Until more satisfactory statistical models become available, it may be prudent to use a non-parametric statistical procedure to determine whether or not two samples, one drawn from the control group and one from the group of treated animals, belong to the same population (null-hypothesis). The rank tests by Mann & Whitney (1947), based on the so-called Wilcoxon Test, seem to be the methods of choice. Correction for tied ranks is possible (Walter, 1951). If more than two independent samples are to be compared, the test described by Kruskal & Wallis (1952) can be used. These tests require that the per animal sample size of cells is constant. From the tables of critical values of the test statistic U, it can be deduced that at least 4 animals in both groups are required before a test ($\underline{P}$ = 0.05) can be applied.

Data from control animals should be tested for inhomogeneity by means of the binomial dispersion test (Snedecor & Cochran, 1967) and should only be accepted if homogeneity is obtained. In experimental groups, individual animal response to the treatment may vary such that inhomogeneity is obtained. Therefore, standard deviations should be calculated with the sample size given according to the number of animals and not the total number of cells scored.

For micronuclei in mouse bone marrow, the spontaneous rate in the controls is 0.2% and fairly constant. Scoring 2000 polychromatic erythrocytes per animal, 1000 per slide, has proved practical, but is still an arbitrary value. Likewise, the spontaneous frequency of breaks in mouse bone-marrow metaphases is 0.5 - 1.0%, and the arbitrarily chosen number of cells to be scored per animal is 125. Practical experience with known clastogens has shown that, using these samples with 4 animals per group, significant differences can be recognized by the rank test if the experimental value is twice as high as the control value, i.e., the spontaneous rate is doubled.

2.8.4   Discussion

2.8.4.1   Possible errors in microscopic evaluation

Microscopic evaluation of metaphase chromosomes for chromosomal aberrations is somewhat subjective. The criteria for the discrimination between gaps and breaks, for instance, has been discussed frequently, and two general opinions exist:

(a)   A gap is an unstained region in the chromatid that is smaller than the width of the chromatid. If the unstained region is larger, it is termed a break.

(b)   An unstained region in the chromatid is termed a gap if no dislocation of the fragment is recognizable. The length of the unstained region is not important. The dislocation characterizes the break.

As discussed in the introduction, it is generally believed that, unlike breaks, gaps do not represent true discontinuities with DNA. This view suggests that the second criterion should be chosen. Opinions differ, however; for example, Scott et al. (1983) recommend the first criterion.

Another subjective element is the choice of analysable metaphases, particularly as the loss of chromatid alignment can contribute to failures in the recognition of aberrations of the chromatid type.

Mouse chromosomes carry a heterochromatic region near to the centromere. Often, the centromeres appear separated from the rest of the chromatids, and this separation may be more pronounced in one chromatid than in the other. This phenomenon should not be mistaken for a gap. Quite frequently, two acrocentric mouse chromosomes may appear in close juxtaposition at their centromeric ends and, thus, mimic a Robertsonian translocation. True centromeric fusions to Robertsonian translocations are very rare events. Chromatid breaks in the centromeric region lead to whole arm exchanges, which should be clearly distinguished from short-arm association due to preparational artifacts.

It is important that only cells with the complete number of centromeres are included in the scores. If cells carrying an aberration, but lacking some of the chromosomes, were included in the scoring, it would be biased in favour of aberration-carrying cells. If normal cells with one or two fewer chromosomes were included in the scores, it would be biased against aberrations, since the lost chromosomes might have been aberrant.

Artifacts can also obscure the micronucleus scores. Granules shed by mast cells have already been described. If they lie on PCEs, they can be mistaken for micronuclei. Granular or fibrillar structures in or on PCEs can be discriminated from micronuclei by their irregular appearance. True micronuclei are round or, on rare occasions, oval or half-moon shaped, but always with a sharp contour and evenly stained. Most artifacts can be recognized as such by focusing up and down. If the particles show a ring of reflection when out of focus, they are artifacts.

2.8.4.2 Comparison of test sensitivity

The two methods, metaphase analysis and micronucleus test, are described, in most cases, as if they were equally sensitive. Accumulating evidence supports the theoretical expectation that metaphase analysis is more sensitive (Kliesch & Adler, 1983). It is certainly more time consuming. However, it should also be more exact, because all types of aberrations are scored. As stated earlier, micronuclei reflect basically acentric fragments. Equating the frequency of acentric fragments at metaphase with the frequency of micronuclei in simultaneous experiments demonstrated that, for an expected frequency of micronuclei, the observed micronucleus frequencies were always below the expected, but without any particular pattern of reduction. Thus, it has to be assumed that not every fragment forms a micronucleus. Other possibilities are that it can be maintained in the main nucleus, or that it can be lost from observation because of cell death. Furthermore, the micronucleus, as such, can be expelled with the main nucleus. On the other hand, the micronucleus test can reveal chemicals that disturb the function of the spindle, such as colchicine or related spindle poisons, or chemicals that predominantly act on tubular proteins rather than DNA, thus inducing aneuploidy instead of structural chromosomal aberrations. For the reasons mentioned above, the two tests cannot be regarded as true alternatives. Thus, even though metaphase analysis requires a higher degree of skill and is more time consuming than the micronucleus test, the extra effort would seem justified.

2.8.4.3 Application of the method to other tissues

Chromosomal aberrations can be evaluated in most tissues of treated experimental animals, whether somatic or germinal, e.g., lymphocytes, spleen, or liver (after stimulation by partial hepatectomy or in vitro) (Dean, 1969), ascites tumours (Adler, 1970), early cleavage stages of embryos (Brewen et al., 1975), embryonic tissues (Adler, 1981), spermatogonial mitoses (Adler, 1974), and meioses of spermatocytes and oocytes (Adler, 1982; Adler & Brewen, 1982). However, because of the increased effort needed to examine the preparations, the use of these tissues is, at present, confined to special studies.

Similarly, micronuclei can be counted in the cells of various tissues, despite the presence of the main nucleus. Reports on the application of the micronucleus test to rat liver hetaptocytes (Tates et al., 1980), mouse embryonic liver and blood erythrocytes (Cole et al., 1979), and rat spermatids (Lähdetie & Parvinen, 1981) have been published.

2.8.5 Conclusions

It is frequently stated that in vivo methods lack the necessary sensitivity compared with in vitro studies. This argument is more than offset by the considerable advantage that an in vivo study is much closer to the human situation, which is the ultimate concern of these studies. In vivo metabolic processes such as activation and detoxification have to be stimulated in vitro by relatively crude enzymatic preparations. Thus, negative results in vivo may be more relevant than positive results in vitro, even with mammalian cell preparations. The resolution of these discrepancies requires careful additional studies on the metabolism of the chemical. Whether the problem is resolved depends on an understanding of whether or not the test compound or one of its metabolites reaches a target organ in significant amounts and what is the half life of the molecule at the target site. It is also necessary to establish that the same metabolite occurs in the in vitro and in vivo situation. If similar

information can be obtained from studies on human beings, then
sound grounds for a decision on whether or not a particular
agent poses a genotoxic danger have been established.

2.9   Dominant Lethal Assay

2.9.1   Introduction

The term dominant lethal is used to describe a genetic
change in a gamete that kills the conceptus early in
development. Any induced changes that affect the viability of
the germ cells themselves or render the gametes incapable of
participating in fertilization are excluded. The pioneering
studies of Hertwig (1935), Brenneke (1937), and Schaefer
(1939) had already indicated that litters sired during the
pre-sterile period of irradiated male mice were found to be of
reduced size. Since there was no effect on sperm mobility and
since the number of fertilized eggs was normal, it was
concluded that the reduced litter size was due to death of
embryos after ferilization. The observation of various
nuclear and chromosomal abnormalities in fertilized ova led to
the conclusion that embryonic death was caused by chromosomal
abnormalities, induced by irradiation in spermatozoa. The
dominant lethal assay was used as an indicator of
radiation-induced mutations by Kaplan & Lyon (1953), W.L.
Russel et al. (1954), and recommended for mutagenicity testing
by Bateman (1966).

To study the cytogenetic basis of chemically-induced
dominant lethals, Brewen et al. (1975) collected fertilized
ova from females mated to young adult male mice after
treatment with methyl methanesulfonate (MMS). The ova were
collected from day 1 to day 23 after injection. The types of
aberrations observed were predominantly double fragments
(presumably isochromatid deletions), chromatid interchanges,
and some chromatid deletions, as well as a shattering effect
of the male chromosomal complement at 100 mg MMS/kg body
weight during the peak sensitivity of dominant lethal
induction. These data strongly suggest that chromosomal
aberrations observed at the first cleavage division of zygotes
are the basis of MMS-induced dominant lethality. In general,
it can be concluded that most dominant lethals probably result
from multiple chromosomal breaks in the germ cells.

A basic problem of chemical mutagenesis is that it is not
possible to measure directly the genetic effects of chemicals
in human germ cells. Therefore, there is no alternative to
using the data obtained in studies with mammals, particularly
the mouse, to predict the induction of mutations in human
beings. The general belief that the human gonads are well
protected (Neel & Schull, 1958) was one important reason for a

20-year delay between the discovery of the induction of mutations by chemicals and the development of research programmes for mutagenicity testing.

The effectiveness of the blood-testis barrier (Setchell, 1970) was sometimes wrongly used as an argument to conclude that the dominant lethal assay is insensitive. In fact, the dominant lethal assay is one of the few test systems that provides information about compounds that are able to cross the blood-testis barrier. Such information is of great importance in the assessment of the possible mutagenic hazard of a chemical.

When a chemical substance has penetrated the blood-testis barrier, it might be subjected to the enzymatic activation processes in the various tissues of the gonad. The compound can also be detoxified. After these modifying processes, the chemicals or their metabolic products may interact with the DNA. The resulting damage may be subjected to different DNA repair processes and, finally, a sperm develop that may or may not carry a mutation. In addition, Generoso et al. (1979) demonstrated that the yield of chemically-induced dominant lethal mutations in male mice depends on the genotype of the female, and this difference between females of different strains may be caused by differences in the activity of the repair enzymes. Though the possibility cannot be ruled out that the induction of a repair enzyme was stimulated by the chromosome lesions themselves, it seems more likely that the repair enzyme existed in the egg prior to sperm entry.

2.9.2   Procedure for male mice

The method consists essentially of sequential mating between treated or untreated male mice and untreated females. Mating usually occurs at night, and conceptions can be recognized the following morning by the presence of a vaginal plug. This plug is a convenient means of timing a pregnancy. Pregnant females are sacrificed on the 14 - 16th day of pregnancy. The corpora lutea, representing the number of ova shed, are counted. The uterine contents are scored for early and late deaths and living fetuses. The induction of dominant lethals is determined by the increase in pre- and postimplantation loss of zygotes in the experimental group over the loss in the control group. This simple procedure is an essential advantage of the dominant lethal assay.

The testis of the adult male contains the complete sequence of maturation stages of the germ cells, from the stem-cell spermatogonia to the spermatozoa passing out of the testis into the epididymis. The timing of this sequence has been determined for the mouse by Oakberg (1960). The earliest time at which specified cells reach the ejaculate is:

1 - 7 days	spermatozoa
8 - 21 days	spermatids
22 - 35 days	spermatocytes
36 - 41 days	differentiated spermatogonia
more than 42 days	A_S (stem cell) spermatogonia.

During the first day after conception, fertilized eggs remain aggregated in the cumulus of follicle cells. By the 4th day, a blastocyst has developed. The blastocyst passes from the oviduct into the uterus. It is the most advanced stage to which a fertilized egg can develop without implantation. Implantation occurs on the 5th day. By the 10th day, organogenesis is complete and, during the following 10 days, the existing structures differentiate, and the embryo completes its development (Bateman & Epstein, 1971). Dominant lethals include the loss of fertilized eggs before and after implantation.

The various germ-cell stages have different sensitivities to the induction of dominant lethals by chemical mutagens, and the germ-cell stage assayed depends on the interval between treatment and mating. The frequency of dominant lethals can change drastically in a 24-h mating interval (Ehling et al., 1968). Therefore, it is essential to use a sequential mating schedule of only a few days. An overview of the differential induction of dominant lethals has been made by Ehling (1977).

The recommended test systems for mutagenicity screening are generally based on the expertise and the facilities of a given laboratory. The procedure given here for the dominant lethal assay is based on a collaborative study involving 9 laboratories (Ehling et al., 1978). The comparative testing of substances using the same method in several laboratories was designed to identify criteria that are critical for the optimal conduct of the dominant lethal assay. From these studies, it was concluded that, while certain test conditions could be standardized for improving the reproducibility of results obtained in different laboratories, other test conditions were matters for establishment in individual laboratories, depending on preferences and conditions.

2.9.2.1 Standard and test conditions

(a)   The mating period should be short enough to provide information about the action of a chemical mutagen on a specific germ cell-stage. For screening purposes, where high fertilization rates are expected, a 4-day mating period is recommended.

The reason for this recommendation is the 4-day estrous cycle in female mice. In addition, the incidence of conceptions should be approximately equally distributed over all days, and only a few females conceive on days 5, 6, and 7 during a weekly mating period.

(b)   The total test period should cover the whole spermatogenic cycle, i.e., at least 12 consecutive mating intervals of 4 days each. Limiting of the dominant lethal assay to certain "critical" mating periods of high sensitivity is only permissible in repeat tests, or if the parts of gametogenesis concerned, e.g., spermatogoniogenesis or spermatocytogenesis, are known from previous studies.

The reason for this recommendation is that chemicals of unknown mutagenic action can induce mutations in a very specific stage of gametogenesis. After long-term treatment, however, either a 4-day or a 7-day mating interval following treatment can be used (Anderson et al., 1983).

(c)   The preferred ratio of mating is 1 female to each male.

The reason for this recommendation is the high conception rate of females when mated 1:1. In addition, using a 1:1 mating mode, the results of each female can be directly associated with a certain male. However, other mating modes, e.g., 2 females to each male, are widely used and acceptable, providing a highly fertile strain of mice is used (Anderson et al., 1983).

(d)   Dose levels should be calculated in terms of mg/kg body weight. The dose volume is adjusted according to the weight of the animals, and administered by the appropriate route.

(e)   The allocation of the animals to the various treatment groups must be based on a statistically randomized procedure.

(f)   Results obtained from sick animals or those that died during the course of the trial should not be included in the evaluation, but should be reported.

(g)   The sensitivity of the chosen mouse strains should be regularly checked using a standard dose of a known mutagen (section 2.9.2.2, recommendation (b)). The results of these studies should be documented.

2.9.2.2 Test conditions to be established by each investigator

(a)   The following test conditions are matters for the individual laboratory and are based on the experience of the investigator: animal strain, age, and housing conditions. A preliminary mating to check the fertility of the animals may be necessary, and vaginal plug evidence is useful for this purpose. The spontaneous postimplantation losses depend, not only on the genome and the housing conditions, but also on the age of the females. The optimum age for the genotype of females to be used must be determined. This age is characterized by a maximum number of corpora lutea and a minimum postimplantation loss.

(b)   The suitability of an animal strain for the dominant lethal assay has to be confirmed by using known mutagens that produce specific effects at different germ-cell stages. According to experience gained in a coordinated study, the induction of dominant lethals following the intraperitoneal injection of 20 mg MMS/kg body weight or 40 mg cyclophosphamide/kg body weight is an indicator of the suitability of a particular mouse strain.

(c)   If vaginal plug data are not used to determine the timing of the pregnancy, the autopsy of the females is best carried out a fortnight after the middle day of the mating interval.

2.9.3   Dominant lethals in female germ cells

Females are less suitable than males for the screening of potential mutagens. The treatment of a female with a chemical mutagen could interfere with the hormonal status and thereby the competence of the animal to carry pregnancies to full term. The treatment could also interfere with the implantation or affect the cytoplasm of the ovum in such a way that the chances of it being fertilized are reduced or the cleavage divisions interfered with. The mutagen could also affect the ovulation rate. All these factors are extremely important for the interpretation of dominant lethal studies in the female (Bateman & Epstein, 1971). There is also the simple technical point that, while the mutational response of a male can be analysed by mating it with several females at different times, the response of a female can be studied only in a single pregnancy.

However, for some compounds, it may be desirable to test the induction of dominant lethals in female mice. This will necessitate proving that the ova were fertilized. On the basis of this knowledge, Generoso (1969) developed a method for the calculation of the dominant lethal frequency in females.

2.9.4   Data processing and presentation

The number of animals necessary for mutagenicity testing with the dominant lethal assay depends on the genotype of mice and the quality of the animal husbandry. In simulation runs on a computer, the sample sizes have been determined for NMRI-Kisslegg and $(101 \times C3H)F_1$ mice. The data for simulation runs were taken from a total of 7000 untreated control animals. If a type 1 error of a = 0.05 is assumed, together with an equally large type 2 error of B = 0.05, then the sample sizes required for different alternative hypotheses are given in Table 1 (Vollmar, 1977).

Table 1. Samples sizes for dominant lethal assay in the male mouse[a]

Mutagenic effect[b] (%)	Genotype	
	NMRI-Kisslegg	$(101 \times C3H)F_1$
10	70	45
15	27	19
20	22	15

[a] From: Vollmar (1977).
[b] Lowering of the probability that a live implant will arise from an ovulated oocyte by %.

The presentation of the data should contain all the information required to assess the test design and to evaluate the results. The following items should be stated:

number of females paired (absolute);
number of females with implantations (absolute and in %);
number of implantations (absolute and per female);
live implants (absolute and per female); and
dead implants = postimplantation loss (absolute and per female).

In some strains, corpora lutea counts pose difficulties. Since the knowledge of the number of corpora lutea is not absolutely necessary for the evaluation of induced mutagenicity in the dominant lethal assay on male animals, this count can be dispensed with, even though, depending on the quality of the counts, this entails a loss of information. However, for certain methods of evaluation, the corpora lutea count is indispensable. It is also necessary for the dominant lethal assay on female mice, because, for example, of the possibility of induced superovulation (Russell & Russell, 1956).

If the corpora lutea count has been obtained, it should be stated (absolute and per female) as should the preimplantation loss derived from the difference between the number of corpora lutea and the number of implantations (absolute and per female). Although the postimplantation loss is the most important criterion for the dominant lethal assay, calculations of the frequency of dominant lethals should not be based on the rate of postimplantation losses only. Otherwise, a sterile phase, induced by a highly potent mutagen as a result of cytotoxic effects or a 100% preimplantation loss due to a genetic cause (Kratochvilova, 1978), could be overlooked.

The following formal relationship exists between the postimplantation and the preimplantation losses:

$$DI \leq I, \text{ with } I = CL - PL$$

(DI = dead implants = postimplantation loss; I = number of implantations; CL = corpora lutea; PL = preimplantation loss). This means that after a high preimplantation loss, the maximum possible postimplantation loss decreases automatically, since the number of corpora lutea can be assumed to be fixed when the male mice were treated.

The calculation of dominant lethals comprises principally the pre- and postimplantation losses. These losses are expressed as the mean number of live implants per female. A good approximation for the induced dominant lethal frequency can be obtained by using the formula of Ehling et al. (1968), which is based on the number of live implants:

Frequency of dominant lethals (F_L) =

$$1 - \frac{\text{live implants per female of the test group}}{\text{live implants per female of the control group}}$$

or the percentage of the dominant lethals ($F_L\%$) =

$$1 - \frac{\text{live implants per female of the test group}}{\text{live implants per female of the control group}} \times 100$$

This formula has the advantage that the spontaneous lethal rate, which is independent of the treatment and is specific for each mouse strain, is eliminated so that the proportion of lethals induced by the treatment is directly evident. In addition, if the treatment is effective, this calculation should give a zero value, but the sample size will result in statistically-insignificant deviation from zero in positive and negative directions. The minus deviations are a good indicator of the biological variability of the sample.

A drawback of this formula is that it is not derived from the individual values of the females and does not incorporate interindividual variability, which is obligatory for statistical analysis. Furthermore, this kind of computation presupposes a target model with Poisson distribution, which cannot be assumed in every case. It should be noted that the proposed calculation can only be used for the evaluation of treated male mice. The calculation of the induction of dominant lethals in females is based on the numbers of corpora lutea (Russell & Russell, 1956).

For statistical evaluation, it must be decided which biological model is to be used and which statistical criteria are appropriate. For biometric analysis, 5 variables are available at 3 levels (Table 2). All these variables are integer frequencies and must be rated as discrete variates.

The female should be chosen as the sample unit. Prior to the actual analysis for mutagenic effects, the death rate of the male animals (if required) and the fertilization rate of the females (obligatory) must be ascertained. If there is a significant difference between groups, the analysis of any mutagenic action will be limited, and ambiguous conclusions may result.

The Wilcoxon test, modified by Krauth and recommended by Vollmar (1977) is an appropriate procedure for the statistical analysis of the dominant lethal assay. According to Vollmar, fertilization rate is tested by the exact Fisher-Yates test

Table 2. Variables for biometric analysis

Level	Variable	Abbreviation
I	Number of corpora lutea per female	CL
II	Number of implantations per female	I
	Number of preimplantation losses per female	PL
III	Number of live implants per female	LI
	Number of dead implants per female	DI

and the quotients I/CL, LI/CL or DI/CL by a separate linear rank test for each mating interval.

Haseman & Soares (1976) have compared different statistical test procedures by computer simulations of the dominant lethal assay. They concluded that the Chi-squared test, frequently used for the analysis of the dominant lethal data, may seriously exaggerate the level of significance and should not be used. The inappropriateness of the underlying Poisson or binominal models appears to have little effect on the validity of analysis of variance procedures based on transformed fetal death data. It can be concluded that, until a satisfactory parametic model can be established, nonparametic procedures are to be preferred.

2.9.5   Discussion

Two different approaches are used to determine the frequency of dominant lethal mutations in male mice. One is based on postimplantation death, the other on both pre- and postimplantation loss. The index of dominant lethality based on postimplantation death alone was advocated by Bateman (1958), Epstein & Shafner (1968), and Searle & Beechy (1974). Support for this index comes from irradiation experiments in which Searle & Beechey (1974) found that the decrease in implantations per female was mainly due to failure of fertilization. This finding cannot, however, be generalized to apply to chemically-induced dominant lethals. Results of MMS studies clearly demonstrate that 100% preimplantation death of fertilized ova can be observed in the mating interval, 9 - 12 day post-treatment (Kratochvilova, 1978). The postimplantation index underestimates even the frequency of radiation induced dominant lethal mutations, as has already been pointed out by L.B. Russell (1962). Certainly, for the detection of a chemical mutagen, possible underestimation of the mutation frequency should be avoided.

Calculations based on comparisons of treated and control groups with respect to the ratio of living plus recently dead embryos to corpora lutea, used by W.L. Russell et al. (1954), or with respect to the number of live embryos per females (Ehling et al., 1968), include the pre- and postimplantation losses. The disadvantage of such calculations of dominant lethal frequency is that the formula does not differentiate between preimplantation loss and unfertilized ova. However, no formula, by itself, can achieve such a differentiation. For the exact determination of dominant lethal frequency, it is necessary to determine the rate of fertilization of ova (Kratochvilova, 1978). It should be mentioned that a decreased frequency of fertilization is also an indication of a possible hazard.

A critical review of the mutagenicity of 20 selected chemicals in the dominant lethal assay was published by Dean et al. (1981). Approximately 300 publications were scrutinized, and data from 130 of these were selected for inclusion in the review. This report contains a concise tabulation of the most relevant data and a detailed review of each individual chemical including the lowest dose to induce dominant lethals and the highest dose with no significant dominant lethality. The review also contains data for the induction of dominant lethals in rats.

The protocol described in this paper is based on the experience with the mouse. However, the factors that are important for the optimal test procedure are likewise essential for testing dominant lethals in other species. Species differences for estrous cycle and embryonic development have to be taken into account for the adoption of this protocol for other species.

3. LABORATORY FACILITIES AND GOOD LABORATORY PRACTICE

3.1 Introduction

In order to conduct the procedures described in section 2 according to acceptable scientific standards, certain minimum levels of laboratory facilities and equipment are essential. The design of the facilities and their complexity varies with the type of study to be performed but, in all cases, they are governed by the need to ensure adequate control of cleanliness and sterility, safety, and accuracy and reproducibility of experimental results.

The need for national and international authorities to regulate the manufacture, transport, and use of chemical substances has led to the introduction of legislation to control these activities. Included in this legislation are requirements for the toxicological testing of chemicals that, in most cases, include testing for possible mutagenic and carcinogenic hazards. In order to establish acceptable standards of quality and reliability of the toxicological data submitted to the regulatory authorities, various bodies have published codes of Good Laboratory Practice. The application of Good Laboratory Practice (GLP) in genetic toxicology testing laboratories is described in section 3.3.

3.2 Laboratory Facilities and Equipment

Regardless of whether laboratories are designed for conducting only the minimum of in vitro mutagenicity studies or for carrying out an extensive programme of in vitro and in vivo genetic toxicology testing, the same basic principles of laboratory design apply. For example, separate areas should be provided for microbiology, tissue culture, cytogenetics and, where necessary, for Drosophila testing and plant studies. They will usually be situated in the same building and should be conveniently served by a common glassware washing and sterilising facility. Chemistry and biochemistry laboratories should be available nearby to provide analytical support, e.g., for confirming the stability, purity, etc., of test compounds or for conducting associated metabolic studies. Where in vivo studies are to be carried out, animal facilities should either be housed in a different building or, at least, have a separate entrance to that of the microbiology and tissue culture laboratories. Animal-holding rooms may be required in the main laboratory complex for cytogenetic studies and for providing material for microsomal enzyme preparations.

Particular attention should be paid to environmental conditions within the laboratory. Temperature and humidity should be controlled within strictly-defined limits appropriate to the techniques being carried out. Ventilation should be adequate with a given number of air changes, e.g., 8 - 10/h, but draughts and direct-intake of external unfiltered air should be avoided to minimize the introduction of dust and contaminating microorganisms.

The design of individual laboratories should be based on the provision of adequate bench space for the number of staff to be employed and adequate room for the equipment and storage of materials. The safety of staff should be a prime consideration. Access to areas where studies are conducted should be limited to those directly involved in the testing. Staff should be fully aware of the hazards of working with carcinogenic and mutagenic chemicals, particularly with the safe disposal of chemical waste, and appropriate safety cabinets, protective clothing, and washing facilities should be provided. Such practices as mouth-pipetting should be prohibited, and an area should be specifically designated for weighing mutagens and carcinogens and for the preparation of stock solutions. A high standard of cleanliness should be encouraged in all working areas, and the design of working surfaces, storage areas, ventilation systems, etc., should be aimed at making clean and sterile working practices an easily-attainable objective.

Certain items of equipment are common to most types of testing laboratories. Refrigerators should be capable of safe storage of flammable solvents, while deep freezes are required to be suitable for the long-term storage of materials at low temperature (-70 °C). In areas where the main electricity supply is unreliable, some form of emergency power generation is advisable. A competent glassware washing and sterilizing facility is essential for experimental work of acceptable quality. In addition to properly-trained personnel, a supply of high-quality distilled water and a suitable non-residual detergent are necessary to provide clean glassware. Equipment such as autoclaves and hot-air sterilizers should be of a design appropriate to the types of materials being sterilized.

3.2.1 Microbial laboratories

Two important factors in the design of laboratories for bacterial or yeast assays are the prevention of contamination of cultures by other microorganisms and the protection of staff against exposure to hazardous test chemicals. Experimental procedures should be conducted in appropriate biological safety cabinets in which a curtain of filter-sterilised air protects the worker from chemical exposure and the cultures from contamination. Air from the cabinets should be extracted outside the building through appropriate filters to prevent environmental contamination. Incubators should have precise temperature control, and those used for testing purposes should be in an area where the ventilation system removes any hazardous vapours from volatile test chemicals, when incubator doors are opened. Culture media may be either purchased as ready-poured plates or prepared in the laboratory from basic ingredients. In the latter case, a clean working area must be available for pouring and drying plates. Either manual or electronic devices are available for counting bacterial colonies. A safe means of disposal of cultures should be provided, e.g., they should be sealed in plastic or paper sacks in the laboratory and then incincerated.

3.2.2   Tissue culture laboratories

Laboratories involved in cell and tissue culture are even more dependent on sterile procedures and working conditions than microbial laboratories. Even a small initial microbial contamination can rapidly spread to other cultures and easily destroy a number of experiments and many weeks work. Although the incorporation of antibiotics into the culture medium serves to limit many bacterial infections; contamination with yeast and fungi presents serious problems in inadequate working conditions. The incidence of contamination can be significantly reduced by conducting all manipulations of cell cultures in appropriate biological cabinets. Culture media can be purchased in a ready-prepared form or can be prepared and filter-sterilized in the laboratory. Liquid nitrogen storage flasks are necessary for keeping stocks of cell lines. For many types of experiments, cells are cultured in Petri-type dishes and incubators in which a 5% carbon dioxide (CO_2) atmosphere can be maintained are required. The safety precautions described above (section 3.2, 3.2.1) for handling and disposing of material containing hazardous chemicals also apply to tissue culture procedures.

3.2.3   Facilities for other procedures

The main requirement for cytogenetic studies on mammalian cells or plant material is for high magnification and resolution microscopes with good quality lenses. Microphotography equipment is useful for recording purposes, and a dark-room facility is required for unscheduled DNA synthesis studies.

One of the major advantages of test systems using plants is that many of them can be performed with relatively simple facilities and equipment. For example, root tip chromosome studies in _Allium_ bulbs require little more than a thermostatically controlled water bath, basic glassware, and a suitable microscope, while seeds of _Vicia, Hordeum_, and _Allium_ can be germinated on moist filter paper or in a suitable aqueous medium (section 2.6). Specific locus studies in species such as _Tradescantia_, _Zea_, and _Hordeum_ can be conducted either in controlled environmental chambers, conventional greenhouses or, where climatic conditions are suitable, outdoors. In these cases, some form of control over temperature, light conditions, and humidity is important.

In general, _Drosophila_ studies, also, only require relatively simple equipment. Stock cultures are maintained in glass bottles, smaller vials are used for the experimental procedures, and they need to be kept in a constant temperature room. A means of anaesthetising the flies is required; examinations are carried out using a low power microscope, and it is useful to have a separate area for the preparation of _Drosophila_ medium.

The maintenance of laboratory animal facilities for breeding and experimentation purposes is an extremely expensive part of a toxicology laboratory, and it is probably uneconomical to maintain breeding colonies of rodents wholly for use in _in vivo_ genotoxicity studies. They are usually available from adjoining conventional toxicology laboratories or from commercial suppliers. An animal-holding area to house animals during dosing and dissection is useful for cytogenetic studies, but should be isolated from laboratories undertaking sterile procedures. In addition, the area used for dosing and holding animals during studies should be of a design suitable for housing in safety, animals dosed with genotoxic chemicals. Dominant lethal studies require more extensive animal facilities and should be conducted in a conventional toxicology animal unit.

3.3 Good Laboratory Practice in Genetic Toxicology

3.3.1 Origins and nature of GLP

In the years following 1970, several national governments enacted legislation to control the way in which chemical substances were manufactured, traded, and used. In general, the laws placed the responsibility of testing chemicals to detect potential hazards for man and the environment on the manufacturers, as a prerequisite of their being allowed to market the chemicals. The present-day codes of Good Laboratory Practice (GLP) have arisen as a result of these enactments.

The reliability of the data was of crucial importance to the governmental agencies charged with administering these regulations, and with assessing the risks on the basis of the experimental evidence submitted to them. The US Food and Drug Administration (US FDA) reacted to finding that some of the data being presented were of poor quality and unreliable by publishing a code of practice (Federal Register, 1978), to which all laboratories generating data for submission to this authority were expected to adhere. Conformity with the code was to be monitored by inspectors from the US FDA. Other regulatory authorities, similarly placed, followed in promulgating codes of their own. These authorities included the US Environmental Protection Agency, concerned separately with industrial chemicals and with pesticides, and a number of departments of other national governments.

Trade in chemicals is international and the proliferation of national and departmental codes reflecting different criteria for the acceptability of data would have hindered it. Thus, the work of the Organisation of Economic Cooperation and Development (OECD) in developing its Principles of Good Laboratory Practice in May 1981 (OECD, 1982) was significant as one element in a programme to enable the mutual acceptance of experimental data among the member nations. The OECD Principles are generic, i.e., they are intended to be applied irrespective of the end-use proposed for the material being tested (e.g., drug, pesticide, or industrial chemical) and of the nature of the data being sought (e.g., determination of mammalian toxicity, or of ecotoxicity). Mutual acceptability of study data would also depend on the studies having been conducted in accordance with the OECD Test Guidelines (standards relating to the scientific content of the tests) and on the testing laboratory having been subject to inspection, in accordance with OECD recommendations, by its national inspectorate. Thus, data generated in one country in compliance with the OECD principles and also subject to the other criteria mentioned, should be accepted by all the member states.

Acceptance and recommendation of the Principles of GLP established by the Council of the OECD is not legally binding for the member countries. The various regulatory authorities, within their own countries, are subject to different legislative and administrative systems. The OECD Principles have therefore to be seen as guidelines to be incorporated by each country into its own legislation and adapted according to its special needs. To date, this has been the case when countries or regulatory bodies have issued definitive codes of GLP. However, differences in requirements reflected in existing codes of GLP are not serious, and there is a consensus that adherence to the OECD Principles would ensure the integrity of experimental data. The US FDA rules (US FDA, 1979, 1982) remain the most comprehensively documented of the existing codes.

GLP sets a standard for the management of scientific experimentation so that laboratory management and scientists are able to assure, and regulatory authorities to assess, the integrity and quality of the data generated. As defined by the OECD, it is concerned "with the organisational processes and environmental conditions under which laboratory studies are planned, performed, monitored, recorded and reported". Owing to their origin, codes of GLP relate only to studies made for regulatory submission. Although several codes of GLP exist, the underlying concepts are common to them all; moreover, scientists will recognize that the majority of the requirements are those that have traditionally been regarded as the basis of all sound scientific investigation.

The objectives of GLP are met by ensuring that:

(a) responsibilities of personnel are properly delineated and assigned;

(b) appropriate standards are defined for all resources (staff, facilities, equipment, materials) and for the conduct of work, and appropriate plans are defined for studies; adherence to the set standards and plans is monitored; and

(c) all relevant aspects of the running of a testing laboratory or the conduct of a study are documented and the records are kept so that a study can be reconstructed and assessed in retrospect.

It is worth emphasising the importance of adequate documentation in GLP.

A testing laboratory generating data for submission to regulatory authorities must therefore establish formal systems for fulfilling the requirements of GLP and must document these systems. The salient points of GLP are described and commented on in the following section. More detailed accounts can be found in the Federal Register (1978, 1983), US FDA (1979, 1982), and OECD (1982).

3.3.2   GLP requirements

(a)   Roles and responsibilities of personnel

Three principal and distinct roles can be discerned in relation to the conduct of studies under GLP.

The Management of a testing laboratory carries the ultimate responsibility for running the laboratory and ensuring that compliance with GLP is maintained throughout. Management defines the appropriate standards for all necessary resources including laboratory facilities, equipment and supplies, personnel, and methodologies, and ensures their timely and adequate provision. A particular obligation of management is to appoint a Study Director for each study, before the study starts, and to replace him promptly, if necessary.

The Study Director is the "chief scientist" in overall charge of the study. GLP requires this single point of control to avoid ambiguities and conflicting instructions that might arise from a diffusion of the responsibility among more than one individual. The Study Director must agree to the approved protocol or plan of the study and, thereafter, must ensure that the study is carried out in accordance with the protocol and with GLP. He must obtain authorization for, and document, all necessary deviations from the protocol. He is responsible overall for the technical conduct of the study and the recording, interpretation, and reporting of the observations including unanticipated responses or relevant unforeseen circumstances. The scientist appointed Study Director must have training and experience appropriate to, and commensurate with, his role in the study.

The third principal role identified in GLP is that of the Quality Assurance Unit (QAU). This is a concept adopted from the more traditional and familiar function of product quality control in industry. The "product" of a testing laboratory consists of the data that arise from its studies and the concern of the QAU is with the authenticity and integrity of these data.

The primary responsibility of the QAU is to monitor, by direct observation, the operation of the testing laboratory and the conduct of studies, to ensure that these comply with the approved standards and with GLP and, in the case of the study, that the protocol is being followed. Thus, the QAU must carry out periodic inspections of the facilities and equipment, the operation of the relevant administrative systems and the actual conduct of the experimental work. Surveillance of a study by the QAU must include an audit of the final report. The findings of the QAU inspections or audits are reported to Laboratory Management and, in respect of studies, also, to the Study Director so that necessary corrective action can be taken. It has been the policy of regulatory authorities, when monitoring laboratories for GLP compliance, not to look at the reports of QAU inspections in order to promote the frankness and hence the effectiveness of the laboratories internal monitoring. The QAU must maintain a "master schedule" giving details of the identity and current status of studies conducted at the laboratory.

Personnel of the QAU report to management. They must be entirely independent of staff engaged in carrying out the study that is being monitored, i.e., they may not participate technically and may not be subordinates of the Study Director (it follows that the chief manager of a testing laboratory may not himself be a Study Director). However, the QAU staff need not be dedicated solely to the quality assurance role, e.g., a scientist participating in one study can be assigned quality assurance responsibilities in respect of another. If this expedient is used, the quality assurance documentation must still be kept in the one place in the testing laboratory. QAU personnel must be familiar with GLP requirements and also be knowledgeable about the tests being monitored, though the quality assurance function does not extend to a scientific appraisal of the study and its results.

All staff concerned with studies must have qualifications, training, and experience appropriate to the function to which they have been assigned. This should not only be in respect of the scientific discipline within which their contribution is made, but also in respect of the requirements of GLP. When necessary, appropriate training must be given, the level of which should take into consideration the degree of supervision of the staff member. The management of a testing laboratory must maintain a current job description for every staff member together with a summary of any training and experience received in relation to the job.

(b) Facilities

Laboratory accommodation must be of adequate size and be suitably constructed and located for the experimental work that is to be performed. In genotoxicity work, the safe containment of hazardous materials, both chemical and biological, is an important consideration but, generally, the requirements of personnel safety are prescribed in legislation other than that of GLP. Two criteria are of particular relevance to GLP. First, similar materials from different studies must be sufficiently separated so that no confusion between them can occur. Disciplined working methods, e.g., adequate labelling of containers, will complement, but cannot replace, adequate provision of bench space or incubator capacity to achieve this. However, once laboratory facilities have been provided, foresight is essential to avoid having too many studies at the same stage simultaneously.

Different phases of studies must also be adequately separated to prevent interference between them. Thus, areas devoted to chemistry and formulation, where the test and control substances are handled at high concentrations, should be separate from areas where these materials are encountered at only low concentrations. In the construction of laboratories, appropriate attention should be given to ventilation and access so that the likelihood of cross-contamination is minimized.

Similarly, separate areas are necessary for the storage of contaminated glassware pending its disposal or cleaning. GLP also requires appropriate areas to be made available for administration, e.g., for "writing up", and further areas for the general convenience of personnel such as for changing into and from protective clothing. The requirement for archive space is noted below.

(c) Equipment

Use of equipment that is inappropriate, inadequately designed, or faulty can lead to the generation of unreliable data. Furthermore, equipment must be properly maintained and, where relevant, calibrated. It should, therefore, be easily accessible for inspection, cleaning, and servicing. These rules apply both to equipment used to generate data (laboratory instrumentation) and equipment used to maintain special environmental conditions.

Written instructions, i.e., Standard Operating Procedures (SOPs) (see below), must be provided concerning procedures for the use, cleaning, and routine care of the equipment. These should include schedules for the items of routine maintenance and the name of the person responsible for seeing that they are carried out. Appropriate action in the event of breakdown must also be covered. Much of this information will be available in the manufacturer's literature, but, where necessary, the handbook must be supplemented, e.g., to cover variations in technique peculiar to the laboratory. This documentation must be freely accessible in the area where the equipment is used.

Written records must be kept of all routine maintenance of the equipment and also of non-routine events such as repairs after breakdown. In the latter case, the nature and circumstances of the defect and the remedial action taken must be recorded. \ One instance of equipment malfunction could conceivably affect the data from more than one study. Therefore, while routine equipment maintenance records can be regarded as non-study specific and filed chronologically, individual study records should enable equipment used in the study to be identified and unscheduled events to be noted.

(d) Standard operating procedures (SOP)

Under GLP, the routine methods of a testing laboratory, as well as some administrative procedures that relate to the conduct of studies, have also to be documented in the form of "standard operating procedures" (SOPs). Written SOPs serve to ensure that all staff are familiar with, and use, the same working methods; thus, errors or loss of data arising from variability between individuals is minimized. They can serve also as a documented specification of the laboratory's procedures, helping evaluation of study methods, or the monitoring of compliance for quality assurance purposes. Documentation of the following procedures is usually regarded as the minimal requirement:

Test and reference substances	receipt, identification, labelling, handling, sampling, storage; confirming homogeneity of test formulations, stability under test conditions;
Equipment	use, routine maintenance;
Records	coding, indexing, or labelling of studies and study-related material; collection, handling, storage, retrieval of data; report preparation;
Laboratory operations	special environmental conditions, laboratory techniques, preparation of reagents;
Quality assurance	conduct and reporting of inspections/audits; record keeping.

Working methods should be presented in SOPs in sufficient detail to ensure the integrity of study data, judgement of their adequacy being the prerogative of management. The degree of detail should also be such that the SOPs can be understood and followed by trained staff. The instructions should cover any work necessary, preliminary to the main procedure, e.g., methods of sampling prior to the application of a given test, and should extend to procedures for the

handling of data and records. Citation of published
literature is permissible to supplement the text of an SOP.
Copies of both the SOP and any supplementary document cited
must be freely available in the area where the procedure is
carried out.

Adoption of a given standard procedure by a testing
laboratory and any changes made have to be approved by the
laboratory management and all changes must be formally
documented. The laboratory must then retain copies of the
superseded SOPs with a record of the dates of their
implementation and replacement. It has been claimed that too
rigid documentation of standard methods can present
difficulties in scientific areas, such as genetic toxicology,
where techniques are undergoing rapid evolution, but
regulatory authorities have not excluded genotoxicity studies
from the requirement. Deviations (as distinct from
significant changes) from a documented SOP in the course of a
study can be made on the authorisation of the Study Director,
provided that such departures are noted in the experimental
record, if not already anticipated in the study plan.

(e) Planning conduct and monitoring of studies

Sound experimentation requires clear objectives and a
definition of how the objectives are to be attained. The
design and methods of the study can then be evaluated in
relation to its objectives to ensure that attainment of the
latter is within the proposed scope of the study. Few studies
are entirely within the compass of a single scientific
discipline and involvement of all the relevant professionals
at the design stage is highly desirable. For these reasons,
the protocol or plan of a study under GLP must be drawn up in
writing before the study starts. The codes of GLP itemize the
information that the protocol must contain but, fundamentally,
it must state the objectives and, in detail, all of the
experimental design and methods that are to be used. Citation
of readily available documents such as SOPs is in order. The
protocol must be formally approved by the laboratory
management and, where appropriate, by the sponsor of the study
and must be agreed to, and signed by the Study Director. Where
changes in the protocol become necessary during the course of
the study, these must be justified and documented in a formal
protocol amendment, signed by the Study Director. Except as
provided for in protocol amendments, the conduct of the study
must then follow the approved protocol and any inadvertent
derviations must be documented in the experimental record.

The batch or sample indicator, as well as the chemical
identity of the test substance, will be given in the study
protocol and records, but it is also necessary to characterize

the test substance and authenticate the sample by appropriate
chemical tests. In this connection, the stability of the test
substance itself has to be known; moreover, if its stablity
under the test conditions, i.e., in the formulation media, is
not known, exposure of the test organism to the intended
challenge cannot be assured. The homogeneity, concentration,
and stability of the test formulation must therefore be
determined.

In GLP, considerable importance is attached to the
authenticity of the records. Observations and data must be
recorded directly and indelibly, and any changes made to the
original record must not obscure the superseded entry. Each
entry or change must show the identity of the originator and
the date, and the justification for the changes must be
included. The originals of data records, termed the "raw
data", have a special importance in GLP in that they have to
be preserved, though exact copies of the originals are also
acceptable (not, however, expurgated records transcribed from
the originals into clean notebooks.)

The conduct of studies under GLP calls, therefore, for a
disciplined approach to the making and recording of
observations and measurements. Responsibility for the
accuracy and completeness of the data resides formally with
the Study Director, though he is not expected to validate
individual entries; rather, he should assure that recording
methods are adequate. Careful attention to the design of the
data-collection methods, e.g., the provision of printed data
sheets that incorporate prompts to help ensure completeness of
the entries and display them for easy review, can complement
valuably the proper training and supervision of the
operators. However, the correct recording of unanticipated
events or observations must not be overlooked.

The role of the QAU in monitoring the operation of the
laboratory facilities and the conduct of studies has already
been indicated. For repetitive, short studies such as
genotoxicity studies, the formal GLP requirement to inspect
each phase of every study can be satisfied by inspection on a
random sample basis.

(f) Reports

The final report of a study must be a complete
presentation of its objectives, the results of the
observations made, and the conclusions drawn from them. To
enable accurate evaluation of the conclusions to be made, the
conditions under which the work was done must be correctly
described, including unplanned occurrences.

An additional requirement under GLP is that the report
must be audited against the raw data by the QAU. This is to

ensure that the methods and conditions of the study are
correctly given and that the results reported are an accurate
reflection of the raw data recorded. An evaluation of the
interpretations placed on the results by the scientists is
beyond the remit of the QAU. The report must include a
statement signed by the QAU listing the dates on which the
inspections and audits of the quality assurance programme
(including the audit of the report itself) were made and when
the findings were presented to management.

The Study Director must sign and date the final report;
this signifies the termination of the study. Subsequent
changes to the report must be made formally, the amendment and
its justification being signed and dated by the person
responsible.

(g) Archives

Full evaluation of a completed study and its report could
necessitate reconstruction of part or all of the study and
this would require access to the experimental records. A
suitable archive for the preservation of the records must,
therefore, be provided. At the end of a study, the Study
Director must ensure the transfer to the archives of all the
raw data and other relevant documentation as well as the
approved protocol and the final report. Records that are not
specific to any study, such as records of staff training, of
equipment maintenance, and superseded SOPs, will also be
stored in the archive.

Control and care of the archive and its contents must be
vested in a named individual, with access to the archive
restricted to authorised personnel. Storage of the material
must be orderly with appropriate indexing to facilitate its
retrieval. The period of time for which the records of a
given study are retained should be in accordance with the
rules of the regulatory authority to whom a submission based
on the study will be made. This period cannot easily be
predicted but a requirement in excess of ten years should be
anticipated. Reasonable precautions, having regard to the
prevailing risks and climatic conditions, must be taken to
ensure that the stored records remain viable for this period.

3.3.3 Summary of resources and records needed

The resources and mechanisms that must be established and
the records that must be kept to comply with GLP are
summarized in Table 3.

Table 3. Resources and mechanisms that must be established and records that must be kept to comply with GLP

Resource	Provision	Documentation
Personnel	Adequate appropriate staff Study Director Quality Assurance Unit Archivist	Responsibilities Training, experience
Facilities	Laboratories (biological, chemical) Administration/personnel Archives	Special conditions, procedures procedures, indexing
Equipment	Adequate capacity, appropriate design	Methods of use and maintenance Records of maintenance
Methodologies/ administrative systems	Scientific techniques Protocol development, approval Test substance handling, authentication Data collecting handling, storage Quality Assurance	SOPs indexing

Records to be preserved

Personnel responsibilities, training and experience

Equipment maintenance

SOPs: superseded editions, with dates

Experimental records

protocols
"raw data"
reports

Master schedule of studies

Quality assurance reports

4. SELECTION, APPLICATION, AND INTERPRETATION OF SHORT-TERM TESTS

4.1 Introduction

The procedures described in section 2 of this guide are those that are generally accepted as suitable for testing chemicals for mutagenic and putative carcinogenic activity. Some are more widely used than others, and the purpose of this section is to offer practical guidance on the use and interpretation of these tests on the basis of current knowledge, experience, and acceptance. It must be emphasized that there is no universal agreement on the best test or combination of tests for a particular purpose, though there have been attempts to harmonise the selection of the most appropriate assays by national and international bodies such as the Organisation for Economic Cooperation and Development. An expert committee of the International Commission for Protection against Evironmental Mutagens and Carcinogens (ICPEMC) is also considering the question of the most effective combination of short-term tests to detect mutagenic and carcinogenic chemicals. In addition, the International Programme on Chemical Safety has organized a series of international collaborative studies aimed at assessing the performance of short-term tests. The results of the latest of these, the IPCS Collaborative Study of Short-term Tests for Genotoxicity and Carcinogenicity (CSSTT), has recently been published (Ashby et al., 1985).

The objective of testing chemicals in these short-term procedures is to provide an assessment of the possible mutagenic and carcinogenic hazards associated with the release of the chemicals into the human environment. No single test has yet been devised that can achieve this objective with certainty. By the judicious selection of a combination of assays, however, and by strict adherance to certain minimum technical and scientific criteria in their conduct, the possible genotoxic hazard of many groups of chemicals can be assessed with a useful degree of confidence. Such assessments are inevitably subject to errors, varying in magnitude, that are influenced by, among other factors, the suitability of the chosen assays for a particular class of chemicals. Furthermore, assays that detect genotoxic activity do not usually detect tumour promotors, hormones, and various other factors that affect tumour formation.

The possible adverse consequences of human exposure to a specific chemical will rarely be assessed from short-term tests alone. Rather, the judgment is made from a total toxicology data package that may include, depending on the nature of the chemical or product, short- and long-term animal studies including tests for reproductive effects, irritancy, sensitisation, neurotoxicity, and data on the absorption, distribution, metabolism, and excretion of the chemical. Data from some of these studies may also help achieve a proper understanding of the significance of the results of short-term tests.

Following the overall assessment of the possible human hazard from exposure to a chemical, the potential risk associated with human exposure is estimated by a regulatory process called risk management. In this process, the potential hazard is balanced against the likely extent of human exposure, the perceived benefit of using the chemical, and other considerations. Risk management involves non-scientific as well as scientific considerations and should not be confused with hazard assessment, which is based on the scientific evaluation of toxicological data.

4.2 Selection of Assays

Some 20 - 30 diffferent assays are referred to in the eight subsections of section 2. The selection of the most appropriate of these to meet a particular requirement is governed by a number of factors. These include the type of genetic change to be detected, the metabolic capability of the procedure in relation to the structure of the chemical to be tested, the predictive value of the assay in terms of mutagenicity and carcinogenicity, the available expertise and facilities and, when appropriate, the legislative requirements of regulatory authorities.

4.2.1 Detection of the major types of genetic damage

Chemicals that interact with DNA produce lesions that, after the influence of various repair processes, may lead to genetic changes at the gene level, e.g., gene or point mutations, small deletions, mitotic gene conversion (e.g., in yeast), or various microscopically-visible chromosome changes; assays are available to investigate each of these events (section 1).

4.2.1.1 Gene mutations

The most widely used and most fully validated assays for detecting chemically induced gene mutations are those using bacteria (section 2.1). They are relatively simple to perform, reproducible, and give reliable data on the ability of a chemical to interact with DNA and produce mutations. It should be remembered, however, that bacteria are very simple organisms, and that a positive result in a bacterial assay does not necessarily indicate that the compound will induce similar effects in animal cells or other eukaryotes. Likewise, a negative result does not invariably mean that the compound lacks mutagenic activity in eukaryotic cells or in intact mammals.

In order to generate data on gene mutations in eukaryotic cells, a choice of screening test systems is available, including certain procedures with yeasts (section 2.2), cultured mammalian cells (section 2.5), Drosophila (section 2.7) and, to a lesser extent, some plant systems (section 2.6). Each of these has certain advantages and disadvantages that will be further discussed later in this section.

4.2.1.2 Chromosomal damage

As discussed in section 1, chromosomal aberrations are changes in the structure of eukaryotic chromosomes. The simplest assays for investigating clastogenic (i.e., chromosome-breaking) effects are those involving either cultured mammalian cells (section 2.4) or plant root tips (section 2.6). These tests can identify chemicals capable of inducing chromosome damage, per se. In order to investigate the ability of a chemical to produce chromosome damage in the whole mammal, two well-established in vivo procedures are available. Clastogenicity in somatic cells can be studied in the bone-marrow cells of rodents dosed with the suspect chemical, either by counting micronuclei in polychromatic erythrocytes or by analysing chromosomes in metaphase cells (section 2.8). Alternatively, chemicals that cause chromosome damage in germ cells can be detected using the dominant lethal assay (section 2.9).

There is increasing evidence that chemically-induced numerical chromosome changes (i.e., aneuploidy) as well as being the cause of much inherited disease, are associated with the carcinogenic process. Among assays for detecting such chemicals, a system using yeast is described in section 2.2. It is not yet clear, however, how predictive this test is for effects on mammals.

4.2.1.3 DNA damage

Three of the procedures described in section 2 are generally accepted as assays that respond to chemically-induced DNA damage. One cellular response to such damage is the initiation of enzymatic repair of the damage, which involves the synthesis of a new, relatively short, strand of DNA. Such repair, referred to as "unscheduled DNA synthesis" or UDS (to differentiate it from the synthesis occurring during normal cell replication), is the basis of the UDS assay in cultured mammalian cells (section 2.3). Mitotic gene conversion in the yeast Saccharomyces cerevisiae, involves the accurate transfer of small segments of DNA between homologous chromosomes and is also regarded as a useful indicator of primary DNA damage. The investigation of sister chromatid exchange (SCE) in cultured mammalian cells also falls within this category. Although the molecular mechanism of SCE formation has still to be fully elucidated, it has been shown to be different from the mechanism leading to chromosome breakage, and the SCE assay is a useful method for detecting chemicals that interact with and damage DNA.

4.2.2   Scientific validity

Before a short-term test can be used with confidence, it must be shown to be a valid procedure for the purpose of detecting genotoxic chemicals. The target cell of the assay, whether it is a bacterium, a yeast, or an animal cell, must be fully characterized both genetically and biologically to ensure that it will respond in the expected fashion in the experimental system in which it is being used. The second important factor is the experimental system itself. The system must be capable of maintaining the target cell in optimum experimental conditions while ensuring that the test chemical has every opportunity of reaching the molecular target (e.g., DNA) in the cell in its most reactive form. Third, the assay must be shown to be "robust", i.e., it should be fully reproducible so that data generated in different laboratories are comparable.

4.2.2.1 Genetic basis

The genetic basis of the target cells used in the bacterial and yeast assays is described comprehensively in sections 2.1 and 2.2, respectively. Guidance on the maintenance of the genetic integrity of the suggested strains is also given. The details given in these sections must be followed faithfully to ensure that the genetic make-up of the test organisms meets the requirements of the particular assay. For example, the Salmonella strains usually used in bacterial assays respond to different types of mutagens, and the range of strains selected must be capable of detecting these different mutagens, e.g., frame-shift mutagens; base-pair substitution mutagens. Similarly, the yeast strains described in section 2.2 have been specially selected to respond to genetic events and it is essential to confirm that the correct strains are used. Similar principles also apply to <u>Drosophila</u> tests in which properly maintained colonies of the correct strains must be used (section 2.7).

With mammalian-cell assays, the situation is slightly different. The cell types described in section 2 are, in general, selected by tissue culture cloning techniques so that they meet the requirements of the genetic change being investigated. For example, CHO cells, used for cytogenetic assays (section 2.4) are selected and cultured in a way that maintains the integrity of the chromosome complement. Cells used in gene-mutation assays (section 2.5) must be sensitive to a particular type of induced mutation (e.g., at the HGPRT locus), and cultures with a low spontaneous mutation frequency are maintained.

4.2.2.2 <u>Metabolic capability</u>

Many carcinogenic/mutagenic chemicals are not able to interact with DNA until they have undergone some degree of enzyme-mediated biotransformation. In animals, including man, foreign chemicals are subject to a series of modifying enzymic and non-enzymic reactions aimed at detoxifying the chemical and altering it to water-soluble forms suitable for elimination from the body. These enzymic reactions are also capable of activating certain chemicals to reactive molecules that can interact with DNA to produce potentially harmful damage (section 1). The appropriate enzyme systems are usually partially or completely inactive or absent in bacteria, yeasts, and cultured mammalian cell systems and are introduced in the form of an enzyme-rich, cell-free fraction of mammalian liver (section 2.1).

An acceptable <u>in vitro</u> assay must, therefore, be shown to have a metabolic capability appropriate to the chemical class being studied and the experimental conditions must be designed to allow the metabolic activation system to operate at an optimum rate. Guidance on these factors is provided in section 2. Although most mammalian cell types used in <u>in vitro</u> tests retain some endogenous enzyme activity, it is usually too low to activate the majority of carcinogens and such tests are supplemented as described above. Some carcinogens, however, have been shown to be poorly metabolized by the conventional rat liver (S9) microsomal enzyme system, but, under appropriate experimental conditions, can be activated by enzymes endogenous to the cultured cell. Technical modifications necessary to detect this type of chemical usually involve a longer than usual incubation period that allows the compound to be available to endogenous enzymes for 18 - 30 h (Dean, 1985).

4.2.3   Predictive value

The ultimate goal of the short-term tests described in this guide is to identify, with an useful degree of confidence, chemicals that may be hazardous. As will be discussed later in this section, such a goal is approached through a series of stages, each of which leads to an assessment of the activity of the chemical at that stage. Proving the safety of a compound is a much more difficult undertaking, rarely performed, and never based on short-term tests alone. In general, given the limited resources available, it is usual to accept a substance as safe in practice in the absence of evidence to suggest otherwise.

4.2.3.1 Mutagenic activity

The first stage in the evaluation of a chemical is to investigate the ability of the chemical to interact with DNA and produce a detectable change in the genetic material. Bacterial, yeast, plant, Drosophila, and in vitro mammalian cell assays are designed for this purpose. They have a high value in predicting whether a chemical is a bacterial mutagen, is active in yeasts or plants, or can induce genetic damage in insect tissues or isolated animal cells. It cannot be predicted with a high degree of certainty, from these assays alone, whether a chemical will produce mutations in a mammal such as man. To provide an insight into the activity of the chemical in the whole animal, in vivo procedures are used in which the chemical is given to test animals by an appropriate route and some means of detecting genetic changes is applied (e.g., chromosome study in bone-marrow cells, dominant lethal assay, or detection of mutagenic excretory products). The predictive value of these in vivo assays is fairly high when positive results are observed. For example, if a chemical produces chromosome damage in rodent bone marrow it is usually assumed that the chemical could present a human hazard, under particular exposure conditions. Negative findings in a properly conducted chromosome study in rodents are also frequently regarded as indicating a low or negligible human hazard, even with a chemical that induces chromosome changes in cultured cells (de Serres & Ashby, 1981; ICPEMC, 1983a). However, certain chemicals, the effects of which are confined to specific tissues, such as the liver or gut, may not be detected using a bone-marrow assay. For such chemicals, tissue-specific assays are being developed, e.g., unscheduled DNA synthesis in rodent liver (Mirsalis & Butterworth, 1980), and an assay for nuclear anomalies in gut tissue (Heddle et al., 1982). There are few practicable procedures for investigating gene mutations in animals and a negative bone-marrow study may have poor predictive value for chemicals that have been shown to induce only gene mutations in in vitro studies. These problems of interpretation are discussed further in section 4.5.

The hazards associated with exposure to genotoxic chemicals differ according to the cell type in which the genetic damage is induced. Mutations in somatic cells are generally regarded as presenting a hazard (e.g., carcinogenic) only to the individual in which they occur. Germ-cell mutations, however, may have far-reaching effects in future generations and it is important to be able to predict whether a mutagenic chemical may present this hazard. Unfortunately, the only practicable procedures currently available for studying germ-cell genetic changes directly are limited to chromosome damage. It is usually assumed, in the absence of evidence to the contrary, that chemicals shown to induce chromosome damage in mammalian germ cells may be able to cause mutations in human germ cells. Negative results in such assays with a chemical shown to be a clastogen in other tests may also be highly relevant (section 4.5). Existing procedures, with the exception of large-scale experimental animal studies such as specific locus tests (section 1) cannot be extrapolated directly to the induction of gene mutations in human germ cells.

4.2.3.2 Carcinogenic activity

As outlined in the Introduction (section 1), carcinogenesis induced by genotoxic agents is a multi-stage process that includes transport and metabolism of the chemical, interaction with the critical target molecule (e.g., DNA), DNA repair and replication of the lesion, and progressive development of the fixed lesion to form a malignant cell. Long-term studies for carcinogenicity in experimental animals do not necessarily reflect a realistic situation as they only measure the ability of a test compound to function as a complete carcinogen. In reality, a person may be exposed to a combination of agents acting on different stages of the carcinogenic process. Current in vitro tests cannot, of course, mimic all these stages and are frequently assumed to detect only the event leading to the initiation phase, i.e., the ability to induce a mutagenic or clastogenic DNA lesion. The main value of short-term tests, therefore, lies in their ability to identify chemicals that may, under certain exposure conditions, either cause cancer by a predominantly genotoxic mechanism or induce the initial phase of the carcinogenic process. Carcinogenesis enhancers (Clayson, 1981), including the so-called tumour promotors, will usually escape detection in the conventional DNA-based assays. It is apparent, from the complexity of the carcinogenic process compared with the relative simplicity of short-term in vitro assays, that, although such assays provide useful qualitative information, considerable caution is required in their interpretation in terms of human carcinogenicity. The predictivity of the tests for detecting potential carcinogens is usually derived from their performance in validation studies in which a range of established carcinogenic and non-carcinogenic chemicals are tested under controlled conditions (the designation "carcinogen" or "non-carcinogen" is obtained from long-term studies in laboratory animals or, more rarely, from human epidemiology data). For example, the predictive value of the Salmonella/microsomal bacterial assay (section 2.1) has been evaluated on a number of occasions, and the accuracy with which it differentiates between carcinogens and non-carcinogens varies between about 60 and 90% depending, among other factors, on the nature of the chemicals selected for the study (Rinkus & Legator, 1979). Technical factors also contribute towards its accuracy and it is important when considering data from bacterial assays (and other tests) that the experimental protocol was appropriate to the chemical type being tested (section 2.3.3). However, a properly-conducted bacterial-mutation assay can give results of a useful predictive value, when considered together with results from other tests.

The induction of structural chromosome damage is also a property common to many carcinogenic chemicals (de Serres & Ashby, 1981), and recent studies have shown that some carcinogens that do not induce mutations in bacterial systems are capable of causing chromosomal damage in cultured mammalian cells (Dean, 1985). Thus, as will be discussed in section 4.5, a combination of a bacterial mutation test and a chromosome assay in cultured cells is considered, by many, to have a higher predictive value for carcinogenic activity than either test alone (e.g., Ashby et al., 1985).

Assays that indicate DNA damage, such as the yeast assay for mitotic gene conversion (section 2.3), SCE in animal cells (section 2.4), and unscheduled DNA synthesis have also provided valuable predictive information on carcinogenic potential. Positive results in these assays generally indicate that a chemical can interact with DNA in a eukaryotic cell, though they do not prove whether or not the lesion induced is capable of progression to a true somatic mutation or a carcinogenic initiation event. Such assays, however, provide useful supplementary evidence in constructing an overall genotoxic profile of the possible adverse effects of a chemical.

Because of the physiological and genetic differences between bacterial and eukaryotic cells, it is inevitable that some chemicals will induce gene mutations in bacteria but not in eukaryotes (and occasionally, vice versa). Assays for gene mutations in mammalian cells (section 2.5), yeasts (section 2.2), and recessive lethal mutations in Drosophila (section 2.7) are extremely useful for detecting some classes of chemical carcinogens.

4.2.3.3 Relevance to chemical class

The experimental protocols outlined in section 2 were designed to provide optimum experimental conditions for testing most types of chemicals. Because of variation in chemical structure and reactivity, it must be accepted that such protocols, particularly for the in vitro tests, are, in reality, compromises, and that, in many cases, the conditions are not necessarily the best for the particular chemical being studied. The nature and rate of the enzymic reactions that transform a pro-carcinogenic chemical to its ultimate reactive form are dependant on the structure of the chemical. The enzymes provided by the microsomal fraction usually incorporated into in vitro tests, i.e., predominantly mixed-function oxidases, are capable of activating most pro-carcinogens. Experimental conditions, including the source (e.g., species, tissue) and quantity of the microsomal fraction and the proportion of co-factors may need to be adjusted to provide near-optimum conditions for a particular chemical class. For example, the standard Salmonella/microsomal assay can detect most aromatic amines, polycyclic hydrocarbons, mono- and bi-functional alkylating agents and mycotoxins, but must be modified to respond to some nitrosamines, metallic salts, and many other compounds. A few compounds, such as 1,2-dichloroethane, are activated by conjugation with glutathione, in which case an exogenous metabolic system may not provide optimum conditions for activation. In addition, compounds activated by enzymes not active in the liver microsomal preparation, e.g., those provided by intestinal flora, will not be detected. These factors apply to all assays that are enriched with exogenous metabolizing enzymes. Other confounding factors may also influence the biotransformation of a pro-carcinogen. For some chemicals, the residual endogenous enzymes in cultured mammalian cells are more active than the added microsomal enzyme mixture (section 4.2.2.2). Under appropriate conditions, the yeast Saccharomyces cerevisiae contains stage-dependant mixed-function oxidase activity that may also be more suitable for the activation of some chemicals.

Although, as already mentioned, the standard protocols for the in vitro assays represent compromises in experimental design, in practice, reliable results can be obtained with most chemicals using these protocols. For the interpretation of results, however, an awareness of the possible influence of the structure of the chemical is an important factor in deciding the adequacy of an experimental protocol for that particular chemical.

4.2.4   Available expertise and facilities

Most short-term test data are generated in government, academic, industrial, or contract laboratories by personnel having considerable experience with the techniques (i.e., section 3). The selection of assays to meet a particular need may, in some respects, be based on the specific areas of expertise and facilities available in a specific institute. For example, a laboratory with a long history of research on Drosophila or fungal genetics may choose to select these organisms in preference to, for example, mammalian cells, for the study of gene mutation. Indeed, in such situations more reliable data might be obtained from these organisms, at least intially, if experience in, or appropriate facilities for, mammalian cell culture techniques were lacking. Similarly, a life-long experience with a particular set of bacterial strains, e.g., Escherichia coli, may lead to their use in preference to Salmonella typhimurium. Although, in principle, some tests have distinct advantages over others for detecting the same type of genetic change, a solid background of experience and an adequately equipped laboratory is essential before attempting to generate data from a "new" (i.e., to the laboratory) assay for hazard assessment purposes.

4.3   Application of Assays

Under ideal circumstances, short-term tests are applied in such a way that, beginning with an initial battery of two to four assays, tests are selected in order to accumulate data on the activity of a compound until a point is reached where an assessment of the probable genotoxic hazard can be made with an acceptable degree of confidence.

4.3.1   The phased approach

Some 80 - 90% of chemicals shown to be carcinogenic in laboratory animals are capable of interacting with DNA and, under appropriate experimental conditions, the majority of assays for mutation will respond to most genotoxic chemical carcinogens. Some assays of genetic damage respond better than others to various classes of chemical carcinogens and mutagens; some carcinogens give consistently negative results in standard assays for mutation-induction, and other chemicals, shown to be non-carcinogenic in laboratory animals are fairly strong mutagens. Since no single assay has proved capable of detecting animal carcinogens with an acceptable level of precision and reproducibility, it is usual practice to apply the assays in "packages" or "batteries". For practical purposes, testing is usually divided into two or three phases or tiers (for review see Williams, 1980), though in many cases, data from the first phase of testing provides sufficient information for a provisional assessment of the genotoxicity of a compound. The first phase, i.e., the basic screen, consists of a battery of two to four assays designed to detect genetic activity in the test material. The second and third phases consist of supplementary assays selected to complement the phase 1 tests, to establish whether genetic damage is induced in vivo and to provide a basis for making an assessment of possible human hazard associated with exposure to the material.

4.3.1.1 Phase 1 - the basic screen

The initial battery (i.e., the basic screen or the "base set") consists of tests with an established broad data base generated from extensive validation studies. One fairly comprehensive package consists of a bacterial mutation assay, an assay for chromosome changes, a test for DNA damage, and a eukaryotic gene-mutation assay. Final selection may be influenced by the nature of the material, e.g., drug, pesticide, industrial chemical, the extent of its eventual distribution and use (section 4.3.2), the objective of testing the material and, in some cases, the available technical expertise in the testing laboratory.

Although a package containing four assays is sometimes recommended for chemicals where extensive human exposure is anticipated (Draper & Griffin, 1980; DHSS, 1981), the assessment of a chemical is often begun with data from an initial battery of just two assays (OECD, 1982b, 1984). These are usually a bacterial assay using a range of tester strains of Salmonella typhimurium (section 2.1) and a test for the induction of structural chromosome aberrations. The latter may be a micronucleus test in rodent bone-marrow cells (section 2.8) or, more often, a chromosome assay in cultured mammalian cells (section 2.4). Providing full consideration is paid to the physical and chemical properties and the metabolic behaviour of test chemicals, few potential mutagens or genotoxic carcinogens will escape detection in a combination of a Salmonella/microsomal activation assay and an in vitro mammalian cell chromosome assay (Ishidate & Odashima, 1977; Ishidate, 1981; Ashby et al., 1985). It must be noted, however, that it is inherent in the concept of in vitro screening that some potentially harmful molecules will slip through the screen and that some molecules active in the in vitro system will prove to be inactive in vivo.

A recent international collaborative study sponsored by the International Programme on Chemical Safety, was designed to identify the assay most suitable to be used in parallel with the Salmonella/microsomal activation assay in a two-test battery for the detection of genotoxic chemicals. Eight carcinogenic chemicals, chosen for the ambiguity of their results in bacterial mutation assays, together with 2 carefully-chosen non-carcinogens, were tested in a variety of in vitro assays (Ashby et al., 1985). A number of assays performed extremely well in differentiating between carcinogens and non-carcinogens in the group of ten. In a final analysis, however, an in vitro mammalian cell culture assay for chromosomal aberrations was selected as the most suitable partner for bacterial tests on the basis of (a) performance in the collaborative study, (b) their advanced state of technical development and wide usage, and (c) a generally internationally accepted broad data base.

It will be evident from the previous paragraph that a reliable bacterial mutation test is widely regarded as a virtually indispensible component of the first phase of testing and that the second test will usually investigate chromosome changes. In some cases, it may be appropriate and more convenient to study the effects of a chemical on chromosome structure in vivo rather than in cultured cells, and assays such as the micronucleus tests (section 2.8) can be used in parallel with the bacterial assay. Though the published data base for in vivo assays is not as extensive as that for cell-culture procedures, the micronucleus test (or a metaphase analysis of bone-marrow cells) has the advantage of using an intact animal and this may provide a sounder basis for hazard assessment. In laboratories where cell culture facilities and laboratory animals are not readily available, it may be necessary to generate chromosome data from plant material. Although well-established techniques are available and a limited number of studies have demonstrated some correlation between plant chromosome changes and mammalian genotoxicity, additional validation of plant systems is essential, before they can be used to assess the potential effects of a chemical on man with any degree of confidence (section 2.6).

As described above, data from a two-test base set can provide reliable detection of most genotoxic chemicals. It must be emphasized, however, that not all chemicals that provoke a positive response in one or both of the tests are necessarily hazardous for man (section 4.5.1). In addition, negative results in these assays do not prove conclusively that the compound lacks genotoxic activity in the intact mammal, including man.

4.3.1.2 Supplementary tests

Supplementary tests are conducted to complement, verify, or assist in the interpretation of the results of the initial battery. They may simply involve repetition of one of the initial assays under different experimental conditions or, in other cases, a completely different type of test.

The results of the basic screen provide information on the ability of the test chemical to induce genotoxic effects in a limited number of assays, e.g., mutation in bacteria and chromosome aberrations in eukaryotic cells. In many instances, these may provide sufficient data and, indeed, may be the only available data on which to make a preliminary hazard assessment. Where, however, a bacterial mutagen does not produce chromosome damage in the mammalian cell assay, it may be useful to know if the genetic activity is confined to bacterial cells, or if the chemical is also active in eukaryotic cells. A variety of systems can be used to answer this question including gene conversion or mutation in yeasts (section 2.2), gene mutation (section 2.5), sister chromatid exchanges (section 2.4) or unscheduled DNA synthesis (section 2.3) in mammalian cells, or mutation in Drosophila (section 2.7). The next stage in the assessment may be to determine whether a chemical shown to be genotoxic in eukaryotic cells is also active in a whole animal. In vitro clastogens can be investigated using chromosome studies on the bone-marrow cells of rodents after dosing with the suspect chemical. The in vivo activity of bacterial mutagens can be further evaluated in studies of mutagenic products in urine or body fluids from animals treated with the compound (section 2.1) (Combes et al., 1984) or in the mouse coat Spot Test (Fahrig, 1977; Russell, 1978). Techniques are also available for investigating DNA repair (Waters et al., 1984) and sister chromatid exchanges (Perry & Thomson, 1984) in treated animals. In some cases, it may be appropriate to study the effect of a compound on mammalian germ cells using either the dominant lethal assay (section 2.8) or chromosome analysis of rodent germ cells (Adler, 1982; Brewen & Preston, 1982; Albanese et al., 1984).

In summary, an assessment of the possible genotoxic hazard is generally carried out after each phase of testing, attempting to answer the questions, a) is the compound mutagenic? (Phase 1); is it active in mammalian cells? (Phases 1 and 2); is it active in vivo? (Phases 2 and 3); does it present a hazard for man? (may be considered after Phase 1, 2 or 3, depending on the nature of the chemical) (sections 4.3.2, 4.5.2).

4.3.2   Nature and extent of potential human exposure

The selection of assays and, in particular, the extent of testing required before assessing the potential hazard, depends on the nature and eventual use of the chemical or product.

4.3.2.1 Limited or negligible distribution

There are chemicals for which environmental distribution is severely limited and the chance of human exposure is unlikely, or limited to small groups of people, the levels of exposure being very low. In these cases, data from a base set of two assays are often the only data available to those who have to determine how such chemicals should be handled. For example, manufacturing intermediates are usually handled by trained personnel using established safe handling procedures and information on the genotoxicity of such chemicals is of value in the design of safe manufacturing processes. Specialized chemicals, that are usually produced in small volumes and supplied for specific industrial or research applications, may be tested in order to assess the safety requirements in their transport or use. For materials of this type, data from both base set assays are normally provided. Only in rare cases is information from a single assay, e.g., a bacterial mutation test, considered adequate, as for example, when screening candidate pharmaceuticals, or dyestuffs, food additives, etc. The results from simple bacterial assays may then be sufficient to identify mutagenic structures in a series of analogues and thus set priorities for further testing or further product development.

4.3.2.2 Medium distribution, limited exposure potential

Chemicals in this group are those to which some degree of human exposure may be possible, but where environmental distribution is restricted and only specific groups of individuals may be inadvertently exposed. Examples include solvents, paints, adhesives, oil products, some pesticides, and other materials that will generally be used in an industrial or commercial environment and to which the general population is unlikely to be exposed. They are chemicals that may be fairly widely used in an environment where potential exposure can be controlled, but do not include materials for domestic use, or those that are present in products available to the general population or are released into the environment.

For assessing the genotoxic hazard of such chemicals, results from two-base set tests together with information on their structural relationship with known carcinogenic and non-carcinogenic chemicals and other basic toxicity data are normally available. Such an assessement may require data from supplementary assays, for example, to confirm negative results provided by the base set or to determine if the genetic damage identified in the in vitro assays can be detected in animals. However, this should not be regarded as a complete evaluation of genetic toxicity.

4.3.2.3 Extensive distribution, intentional or unavoidable exposure

This group contains chemicals, materials, and products that may be widely distributed in the environment and to which human beings will almost certainly be exposed. Examples include: pharmaceutical products, both those used for very specialised treatments and those used by a relatively high proportion of the population; chemicals that are an integral part of foodstuffs or may appear as residues or contaminants in food; domestic and agricultural pesticides; domestic chemicals of all kinds; environmental contaminants including naturally occurring chemicals in plants, soil etc.; combustion products; industrial effluents; and many more.

Because human exposure to these materials is generally to be expected, the objective of short-term tests (and, indeed, of all toxicity testing) is to ensure, as far as possible, that exposure does not present a potential or actual hazard. It is important to keep in mind that the eventual assessment of genotoxicity is aimed at deciding if the chemical presents either a carcinogenic hazard or an adverse effect on germ cells with the possibility of producing heritable genetic damage.

Initially, results of the base set are assessed, but data from these assays are rarely sufficient for hazard assessment for chemicals in this group (section 4.5.1). It is usual to conduct supplementary assays to investigate other genotoxic effects such as the induction of gene mutations or unscheduled DNA synthesis in mammalian cells, and, when this genetic profile has been completed (section 4.5.1.4), to assess the activity of the material in vivo. At this stage, and with the help of data on the absorption, distribution, metabolism, and excretion of the chemical and other toxicological data, it is possible to conduct a reasonable assessment of the potential of a substance for mutagenicity and genotoxic carcinogenicity. The final assessment of carcinogenic potential, however, usually requires the provision of data from long-term cancer studies in laboratory animals.

4.3.3 Regulatory requirements

Many countries require the submission of testing data before approving the marketing of certain types of products. However, the requirements differ considerably between countries, and various national and international bodies have attempted to harmonise mutagenicity testing requirements by preparing guidelines. Organizations such as the Organisation for Economic Cooperation and Development (OECD) and the European Economic Community (EEC) have published regulatory requirements or guidelines for mutagenicity testing, though many countries continue to have their own individual requirements. The specific assays required by individual countries are often unclear and usually depend on the nature of the chemical or product and the outcome of discussions between the marketing company and the competent authority of the country (ICPEMC, 1983b).

Two bodies whose authority extends beyond national boundaries are the OECD (representing some 24 countries) and the EEC. Their guidance and regulations, respectively, on mutagenicity testing are very similar and, in practice, apply to the marketing of new substances rather than existing chemicals. Both authorities relate the extent of testing to the perceived degree of exposure and distribution. For example, testing is only required on chemicals that will be produced or imported in quantities of one tonne or more per annum. Many types of product are excluded by these authorities; medicinal and food products are often regulated by individual countries rather than international bodies.

The OECD and EEC require a base-set of two tests for mutagenicity, i.e., assays for bacterial mutation and for chromosome damage, on all products that are not excluded from their authority, with a requirement for supplementary assays when exposure of relatively large numbers of people is unavoidable or intentional.

4.4 Acceptability and Reliability of Data

It is essential that data used to assess the genotoxicity of a chemical are derived from studies designed to meet predefined minimum technical and scientific criteria. One of the purposes of the descriptions of assays contained in section 2 of this guide is to define these criteria. The reliability of data, therefore, can be confirmed by ensuring that the experimental protocol used to produce the data conforms to the requirements for an acceptable assay. In addition, evidence must be provided to show that the investigator faithfully adhered to the protocol by accurate and full recording of all experimental procedures, raw data, mathematical calculations, etc., so that every step of each assay can be audited by an independent observer. Such monitoring procedures are described in detail in section 3.3.

4.5 Interpretation of Results and Significance for Human Hazard Assessment

Results of short-term tests are assessed with two distinct types of hazard in mind: the carcinogenic activity of the chemical and the possibility that the chemical may affect human germ cells to produce heritable genetic changes.

4.5.1 General principles

Much of the data used in the assessment are generated from relatively simple tests, often consisting of cultures of single cells, and it must be emphasized at the outset that the behaviour of a particular chemical may be dramatically different in a complex organism such as man. In a simple bacterial mutation assay, the chemical may be metabolically transformed by an auxillary microsomal enzyme system and the reactive molecule thus generated has simply to penetrate the bacterial cell wall to be readily available to interact with DNA to produce genetic changes. In the whole animal, however, the same chemical must be absorbed into the body across a number of chemical and physical barriers, and must be transported to the site where the appropriate metabolizing enzymes are situated, where it may be activated or detoxified, before it is in a form that can interact with DNA (some metabolism may also occur in the gut). Even then, the DNA lesion is subject to protective devices, such as DNA repair, before genetic changes are expressed, and these protective factors differ between the bacterial system and animal cells. Thus, in animals, a range of physiological and biochemical factors that are different from those in simple assays may influence the ultimate fate of the chemical, either inhibiting or enhancing its potential toxicity.

The structure of the chemical and its possible fate in animals are important factors in the interpretive process. Data from studies on absorption, distribution, metabolism, and excretion are generally only available for chemicals for which the possibility of human exposure is relatively high, e.g., drugs, foods, and many pesticides, and, even then, detailed metabolic data may not be available. For other materials, the possible _in vivo_ fate may be inferred from the chemical

structure by analogy with related chemicals for which more
information is available.

A further factor in the interpretation of short-term tests
lies in the correlation between positive and negative results
in a particular assay and known carcinogenic and
non-carcinogenic activity. This correlation is obtained from
validation studies in which the activity of known animal
carcinogens and non-carcinogens is established in the
short-term test (Purchase et al., 1978). The assays commonly
used in the initial test batteries, e.g., bacterial mutation
tests and in vitro chromosome assays, are selected because
they have performed well in validation studies and currently
have a good predictive value for animal carcinogenicity with
many classes of chemicals (de Serres & Ashby, 1981; Ashby et
al., 1985).

Thus, the important factors to be considered when
interpreting the findings of short-term tests are: (a) the
predictive value of the assays as demonstrated by their
correlation with known carcinogens and non-carcinogens; (b)
the structure of the chemical in relation to chemicals of
known genotoxicity; (c) the known or probable metabolic route
of the chemical in the whole animal; and (d) data from other
toxicity studies.

In section 4.5.1.1, the significance of the results of
individual assays is discussed, but it must be emphasised that
assessment of human hazard should be based on combinations of
assays rather than on data from single tests. The
interpretation of data from batteries of short-term assays is
described in section 4.5.1.2, together with the application of
the phased approach to assessing genotoxic hazard using
supplementary tests.

4.5.1.1 Results of individual assays

For many years, assays using a range of tester strains of
bacteria have been the cornerstone of short-term tests for
genotoxicity. Positive results indicate, primarily, that the
chemical or one of its metabolites is capable of interacting
with DNA to produce mutations. In spite of the fact that many
genotoxic carcinogens produce mutations in bacteria, not all
bacterial mutagens are animal carcinogens and the
interpretation of bacterial assays in isolation, in terms of
human hazard is not an acceptable procedure. Data from at
least two base set assays are usually available before even a
preliminary extrapolation is attempted, for example, when
establishing safe working practices in a manufacturing plant.

There is increasing evidence, particularly from a recent
collaborative study sponsored by the International Programme
on Chemical Safety (Ashby et al., 1985), that some carcinogens

that are negative or difficult to detect in bacteria induce
genetic changes in eukaryotic systems, such as cultured
mammalian cells, yeasts, or Drosophila, in the form of
structural chromosomal aberrations or gene mutations. Again,
these assays are not usually interpreted in isolation but only
as part of an expanding data base.

Studies on whole animals are usually considered to be more
relevant to man than in vitro assays and, as a general rule, a
chemical that gives clear, unequivocal positive results in an
in vivo assay, such as chromosome damage in rodent bone-marrow
cells or the dominant lethal assay, is usually regarded as a
possible human mutagen or carcinogen.

4.5.1.2 Results from combinations of assays

It is usual practice to begin the assessment of the
genotoxicity of a chemical on the results of an initial
battery of at least two assays. One of these is almost
invariably a bacterial mutation assay and, in a two-test
battery, the second is usually an in vitro or in vivo
chromosome assay. Data from other tests, e.g., yeasts, UDS,
etc., may also be available, and, where other toxicity or
pharmacokinetic studies have been conducted, the data base is
considered as a whole during the assessment of possible hazard.

The following sequence of assessment procedures is based,
as an example, on data available, initially, from a bacterial
mutation assay and a chromosome assay in cultured mammalian
cells. For the purpose of this exercise, it is assumed that
the data have been generated from reliable and acceptable
protocols (section 4.4).

A.   Chemicals clearly positive in both assays

Such findings demonstrate unequivocally that the chemical
or a metabolic derivative is capable of interacting with DNA
to produce genetic damage in both eukaryotic and prokaryotic
cells. It is thus classified as a genotoxic chemical and,
unless, and until, data from other toxicity studies or
supplementary short-term tests show that it is unlikely to be
active in vivo, it is prudent to regard it as potentially
hazardous for man.

In some instances, chromosome data may be presented from
plant systems rather than mammalian cells, and the same
principles apply. However, it may be appropriate to confirm
the plant data in a mammalian-cell assay or other eukaryote
(e.g., Drosophila or yeast) at an early stage.

It may be prudent to designate a chemical as potentially
hazardous on the basis of these assays and this may indicate
that distribution and human exposure will be restricted. The

potential value of the chemical may be such that further
testing designed either to confirm this assessment or to
determine the extent of the potential hazard may be
worthwhile. By no means will all such chemicals be shown to
be hazardous in subsequent testing. Additional testing may be
aimed at elucidating: (a) the nature of the genetic change
induced by the chemical in mammalian cells; (b) the dependance
of the chemical on metabolic enzyme activation for its genetic
activity; and (c) the behaviour of the chemical and the
genetic damage it induces in the intact mammal.

(i) Positive results only after metabolic activation

Such results indicate that reactive metabolites are
generated by microsomal enzymes, i.e., the compound is an
"activation-dependent" mutagen. As the chemical has been
proved to be a clastogen in vitro, the next step may be to
carry out a chromosome study in bone-marrow cells in rodents
after dosing with the chemical by an appropriate route (e.g.,
oral, intraperitoneal). Either the micronucleus test or
analysis of metaphase chromosomes can be used. If the
chemical is shown to produce chromosome damage in vivo, there
is little to be gained by any further testing and it is
usually regarded as having mutagenic or carcinogenic potential
for man. In rare cases, for example, mutagenic anti-tumour
agents, the benefits of using the drug may outweigh this
potential hazard and it may be useful to conduct a dominant
lethal assay or a cytogenetic analysis of germ cells in
rodents to assess the induction of heritable genetic changes.
Negative results in a properly conducted in vivo study may
alleviate most concern regarding the potential hazard of a
chemical and, with many chemicals, such negative results
suggest that the adverse chromosome effects shown in vitro are
unlikely to occur in the intact animal. (It should be
remembered that, occasionally, a negative result may be
obtained in a bone-marrow chromosome study because the
compound or its reactive metabolite(s) did not reach the
target cell in the bone marrow.) However, the chemical is
still a mutagen and the decision to release it into the
general environment will usually be measured very cautiously
against its possible benefits; further testing may be
judicious. Since sister chromatid exchange or unscheduled DNA
synthesis (UDS) are mechanistically unrelated to chromosome
breakage, it may prove useful to establish the activity of the
chemical in these in vitro assays. If either yields a
positive result, in vivo activity can be investigated by
conducting assays for SCE in bone-marrow cells or UDS in
hepatocyte cultures from treated rodents.

A detailed pharmacokinetic profile of the chemical may be available and could provide evidence on the generation of reactive metabolites in vivo. Such evidence may support the assumption that the chemical is or is not putatively genotoxic for mammals.

(ii) Positive results in the absence of metabolic activation

Chemicals that produce mutations in bacteria without the need for exogenous metabolic activation are either "direct-acting mutagens" or, in rare cases, are activated by bacterial enzymes. Most eukaryotes are capable of some degree of endogenous activation (i.e., without the use of an auxillary metabolizing system) and direct-acting chemicals are usually classified as such on the results of bacterial assays. If there is an indication from the in vitro assays that the incorporation of a metabolic activation system eliminates or significantly reduces the mutagenic activity, then it is possible that the microsomal enzymes serve to detoxify the chemical. Some confirmation of this can be obtained from an in vivo chromosome study, from the results of one of the other in vivo tests for mutagenic activity (A(i)), or from the results of a study of the metabolism of the chemical in vivo. Negative results from a properly conducted in vivo investigation of a direct-acting mutagen usually indicate that it is unlikely to pose a serious carcinogenic hazard.

B. Chemicals that produce gene mutations in bacteria but not chromosome aberrations in mammalian cells

A chemical that produces mutations in bacteria with negative results in the eukaryotic-cell test is classified as a bacterial mutagen. The question then arises as to whether the mutagenic activity is specific to bacterial cells. This may be investigated by applying one or more of the other tests described in section 2. Where mutagenic activity is established in a eukaryotic cell system, interpretation of the data and the need for additional tests follows the procedure outlined in A(i).

Occasionally, chemicals are encountered that produce mutations in bacteria, but are clearly negative in other in vitro tests. The assessment of such findings presents a number of difficulties. Interpretation may be helped by conducting an in vivo cytogenetic assay (in spite of the fact that the in vitro chromosome assay was negative, the absence of chromosome aberrations in a bone marrow study is valuable confirmatory evidence), by testing urine from treated animals for mutagenic activity and by consideration of the pharmacokinetics, the relationship of the structure of the chemical to known genotoxins, and other toxicity data. However, the observation of bacterial mutagenicity may be the only evidence that the compound is genotoxic and a great deal of effort can be expended in trying to elucidate its significance to human hazard. Where other in vitro and in vivo tests fail to reveal mutagenic activity, and where there is no evidence from pharmacokinetic and conventional toxicity studies to suspect possible adverse effects, then the finding of bacterial mutagenic activity in isolation, particularly at high test concentrations, may not constrain the use and distribution of most materials. Certain drugs, food chemicals, and ubiquitous materials have been exempt from this view and their use restricted pending long-term cancer studies in laboratory animals.

C. Chemicals that produce chromosome aberrations in mammalian cells but not mutations in bacteria

This pattern of results raises three important questions:

(a) has the chemical been tested in bacteria under an appropriate range of experimental conditions, e.g., using a preincubation technique, variable levels of metabolic activation (i.e., S9), and using an adequate range of tester strains of bacteria;

(b) can the chemical induce mutations or UDS in cultured cells; and

(c) can the in vitro chromosome damage be reproduced in vivo?

Some chemical carcinogens (e.g., hexamethylphosphoramide) give negative results in bacteria but are clearly mutagenic when tested in mammalian cells (Ashby et al., 1985). It is often useful, therefore, to check the mutagenicity in a mammalian-cell system and if shown to be active, it can be assessed as described in A(i). For small-volume chemicals (section 4.3.2.1), the information that a chemical induces chromosome aberrations may be all that is available to formulate guidance on its use and distribution. Where it is important to determine its activity in vivo, a bone-marrow cytogenetic assay using micronuclei counts or metaphase analysis is the next logical step. Positive results in such a test confirm genotoxic activity in vivo and, in most cases, are interpreted as suggesting a possible hazard for man. Where the induction of chromosome damage in cultured cells is

the only indication of genotoxicity, i.e. where other
short-term tests in cultured mammalian cells are negative,
where there is no evidence of chromosomal damage in animal
studies and other toxicity studies do not show any adverse
effects, the chemical is unlikely to pose a genotoxic hazard
for man. As indicated in section B, certain drugs and food
chemicals may be exempt from this view and long-term animal
studies are desirable before the material is released for
human use.

D. Negative results in both assays

In assessing the significance of negative results in the
basic screen, it is essential to determine whether the results
are a true indication of lack of genotoxic activity by
confirming that the protocols used were appropriate for the
type of material being tested. For example, if the chemical
is volatile, assays must be conducted in sealed vessels to
prevent erroneous negative results caused by evaporation of
the test chemical. Some chemicals, e.g., nitrosamines,
require special experimental conditions to detect mutagenic
activity. The physical and chemical properties of the test
agents and the influence of protocol variables on the
performance of the assays are taken into consideration when
evaluating the significance of negative results in the basic
screen. For many chemicals of limited distribution and
exposure, the provision of reliable evidence of the absence of
mutagenic activity in the two initial assays is frequently
considered to be sufficient grounds for regarding the chemical
as non-genotoxic. Because of the existence of a small class
of genotoxic agents that are not detected in the two initial
assays, it must be accepted that a decision to permit
widespread use and unlimited distribution on the basis of
negative results in these tests carries a significant risk,
and further testing in other assays may be of value.

E. Non-genotoxic carcinogens

The majority of carcinogenic chemicals have demonstrable
genotoxic activity. There are certain classes of chemicals,
including, for example, some metals, organochlorine compounds,
and estrogens, that are known to be carcinogenic in animals
but fail to elicit a positive response in assays for
genotoxicity. There are other compounds that are not in
themselves complete carcinogens, which are able to exacerbate
certain stages of the carcinogenic process (ICPEMC, 1982).
Collectively, these latter compounds are referred to as
carcinogen enhancers (Clayson, 1981). At present, there is no
short-term test that has been sufficiently well validated to

11

be used with confidence to detect non-genotoxic carcinogens and enhancers. Evidence is emerging that some of these chemicals can induce numerical chromosome changes in eukaryotic cells and, in some cases, structural chromosomal aberrations (Ashby et al., 1985) and that they can be detected in modified forms of certain assays for neoplastic transformation (Meyer, 1983). However, these findings require confirmation in further validation studies and it must be accepted that a proportion of this class of chemical will escape detection in current toxicological practice.

F.   Complex mixtures

The principles outlined in this guide apply to chemicals that are pure compounds or relatively simple mixtures, formulations, or solutions. The application of in vitro assays to more complex mixtures, e.g., foods, crude industrial products, etc., may give results that are unreliable because of the influence of such factors as, for example, competition between components in the mixture for enzyme sites in the activation system, presence in the mixture of cytotoxic components that limit adequate testing, and uncertainties regarding the concentrations of mutagenic components. In vitro assays, therefore, must be used and interpreted with caution and, where it is not possible to isolate and identify mutagenic components, the emphasis should be on in vivo testing (although it must be realized that problems similar to those mentioned above may beset whole-animal assays).

4.5.2   Influence of the extent of exposure and distribution

The amount of toxicity testing that a material undergoes before it can be released for specific or general applications or into the environment is decided, to a large extent, by its perceived distribution and the expected pattern of human exposure. For each of the broad groups of materials considered here, evaluation of genotoxic activity is based on the phased approach (section 4.3.1) using as a starting point, data from a two-test base set. It must be remembered that mutagenicity tests provide only part of an overall package of toxicity data that should be available before making a final assessment of human hazard.

This guide is concerned only with hazard assessment and it is not within the objectives of the guide to describe methods for estimating, in quantitative terms, the risk of adverse effects in man following exposure to specific genotoxic chemicals. However, in order to avoid confusion between the terms "hazard" and "risk", brief definitions of risk estimation and risk management are outlined.

(a) Hazard assessment

The assessment of the possible hazard associated with exposure to a genotoxic chemical is a purely scientific process and involves an appraisal of experimental data in order to attempt to predict the possibility and the nature of any adverse effect in man.

(b) Risk estimation

This is the second stage in the evaluation of a product or chemical and is an attempt to derive a quantitative estimate of the risk resulting from the use or release of the material, i.e., the number or frequency of individuals in a population of a given size who may exhibit a given adverse effect (e.g., cancer or heritable mutations) under certain exposure conditions. Risk estimation is almost always an uncertain undertaking. Quantitative data derived from screening tests cannot be used as a basis for predicting the potency of carcinogenic activity in animals or man (For additional details see Bridges et al, 1979; Ehrenberg, 1979; Brusick, 1980; Sankaranarayanan, 1982; ICPEMC, 1983d).

(c) Risk management

While hazard assessment and risk estimation are scientific processes, risk management is a non-scientific decision-making procedure (US NAS, 1983). Risk management attempts to balance the perceived benefit of using or distributing the chemical or product with the risk of adverse effects to individuals or to populations, i.e., a risk-benefit equation. Where the benefits are regarded as great, for example with a new, unique and valuable drug or pesticide, an identifiable and measurable risk may be considered acceptable. In situations where less toxic alternatives with similar benefits are available, the risk associated with the introduction of the new material would normally be unacceptable.

4.5.2.1 Pharmaceutical compounds

With few exceptions, pharmaceutical compounds that show unequivocal mutagenic activity are identified and discarded by the drug company at an early stage of development. Most major companies involved in the development and manufacturing of drugs use a three-stage development regime that includes some toxicity testing at each stage. The first stage is an in-house toxicity screen that is used primarily for the selection of candidate compounds, i.e., those that show promising pharmacological activity, for further development.

Only very limited mutagenicity testing is likely to be conducted at this time, and, in most cases, will consist of a bacterial mutation test. Compounds that show mutagenic activity will frequently be discarded at this early stage. There are exceptions to this rule, for example, where a compound or a group of compounds with unique pharmacological activity may be considered of great potential benefit. Promising candidates eventually reach a stage of development where it is necessary to test their efficacy in human beings. Before these clinical trials, the compounds undergo a second phase of testing, i.e., the pre-clinical trial toxicity screen, the objective of which is to assess the safety of the drug for use in small groups of human volunteers. Assuming that a bacterial assay was conducted in the primary toxicity screen, mutagenicity testing usually consists, initially, of either a test for the induction of chromosome aberrations in cultured cells or an <u>in vivo</u> assay in rodent bone-marrow cells for micronuclei or metaphase chromosome aberrations.

The interpretation of the findings from the initial mutagenicity assays is greatly influenced by the pharmacological and pharmacokinetic data generated during the development of the drug. If clear negative results are obtained with a compound that also shows no indication of interaction with macromolecules such as DNA, then it may be regarded as safe enough, from the point of view of genotoxicity, to proceed to clinical trials. Where there is any doubt about the pharmacokinetics of the drug or its metabolites (as is often the case at this stage of development), i.e., where the possibility of DNA interaction cannot be excluded, then additional testing is indicated. The supplementary tests are aimed at filling in the gaps in the genotoxicity profile. For example, if an analysis of metaphase chromosomes in bone-marrow cells from treated rodents was not part of the initial testing, then this is usually also carried out. Although the chemical failed to induce mutations in bacteria, it may be tested in a mammalian cell assay for gene mutations, or, perhaps, for recessive lethal mutations in <u>Drosophila</u> or gene mutations in yeasts. Other tests that indicate the induction of DNA damage may also provide useful data. The pharmacological data available may also indicate the testing of urine and other body fluids from treated animals for mutagenic activity, using bacterial assays. Where the structure of the chemical indicates that nitrosation products may be formed in the human stomach, tests for the formation of such products and their mutagenicity may be conducted (Kirkland et al., 1984).

Thus, before a pharmaceutical chemical undergoes clinical trials in human volunteers, it is normally shown at least to be incapable of inducing mutations in bacteria and chromosome damage in mammalian cells. Where the structure or the pharmacokinetics of the chemical suggest that genotoxic interactions are conceivable, additional testing will usually include analysis of chromosome aberrations in vivo, eukaryotic assays for primary DNA damage and gene mutations and, where indicated, for chromosome changes in germ cells (e.g., a dominant lethal assay) and for mutagenic metabolites in urine or body fluids of treated animals. Assuming negative findings in these assays and after considering the data from other toxicity studies, the drug may then undergo clinical trials.

Except in the case of, for example, cytostatic or cytotoxic drugs used in the treatment of serious, life-threatening diseases, compounds that are shown to be genotoxic will rarely undergo efficacy studies in man. Where there is sound evidence that a drug, shown to be mutagenic in vitro, is rapidly detoxified in intact animal studies, limited clinical trials may occasionally be justified.

The first two stages of toxicity evaluation are conducted as part of the development programme. After successful clinical trials, a final toxicological evaluation is undertaken before the drug is submitted for registration prior to marketing. Registration is usually a responsibility of a government department in the country in which a marketing permit is sought. The genotoxicity data required for registration vary considerably between individual countries though, in most cases, the assays conducted before clinical studies in human beings comprise a package that is acceptable for registration purposes. Some authorities require data from a very specific series of assays, but, in general, a package that includes properly conducted assays for mutations in bacteria, chromosome aberrations and gene mutations in mammalian cells, and an in vivo test for chromosome aberrations (in somatic and/or germ cells) should satisfy most authorities of the absence of a potential mutagenic hazard providing that there is no contradictory evidence from other toxicity studies.

This package of assays also provides some indication of the carcinogenic hazard. However, for registration and marketing purposes with a new drug, carcinogenicity is almost invariably assessed from animal studies rather than predicted from in vitro assays.

4.5.2.2 Chemical compounds in food

Although this section is primarily concerned with chemicals that are added to natural food products to improve their keeping properties, palatability or appearance, etc., it is pertinent to summarize some other factors that contribute towards the mutagenic activity of food (For review, see

Knudson, 1982). Some edible plants and their fruits contain compounds, e.g., pyrrolizidine alkaloids, flavonoids, etc., that are mutagenic in in vitro assays. A small number are also carcinogenic, but the majority have not yet been tested for carcinogenicity. They are often present in only minute quantities in the plant material and are often destroyed when the plants are cooked or completely detoxified by the gut flora. The contribution of mutagenic food components to human cancer is not known. Another source of potential genotoxicity is the fungal contamination of foods, e.g., aflatoxins in mouldy groundnuts. Food may also contain residues of pesticides, compounds absorbed from packaging materials, and other chemicals. An additional contribution to genotoxic activity can occur during cooking, and it has been demonstrated that pyrolysis products, formed during the cooking of meat and fish at certain temperatures, have significant mutagenic activity. Although dietary factors are known to contribute towards the overall incidence of cancer in man, the part played by naturally occurring mutagens and pyrolysis products in human disease has yet to be established.

Most foods are complex mixtures of many hundreds of compounds and evaluating their genotoxicity is far more difficult than evaluating that of pure chemicals. Because of this, attempts to investigate the genotoxicity of whole foods are usually undertaken using intact animals, including Drosophila. However, the fractionation of foods for mutagenicity testing purposes is currently being explored (Rowland et al., 1984).

Artificial food additives include chemicals that either enhance the natural flavour of foods, improve colour or appearance, or are preservatives added to prevent bacterial spoiling or oxidative degradation of food. Artificial flavouring materials are usually identical in chemical structure to naturally occurring flavourings and are either synthesized or purified extracts from natural sources. A large number of natural and synthetic dyes have been used to improve the appearance of food. Many synthetic dyes have been removed from national and international lists of permitted food colourants because of their mutagenic or carcinogenic activity. Compounds commonly used to preserve foods include sodium nitrite, a weak mutagen in in vitro tests, and antioxidants such as butylated hydroxytoluene (BHT). Although the mutagenicity of nitrite itself is unlikely to present a human hazard, it is able to react with secondary amines in conditions found in the human stomach to form carcinogenic nitrosamines.

The application of short-term tests for genotoxicity to food additives follows the principles outlined earlier. Chemicals proposed for use in foods are usually tested initially in a base set of two assays and those that, for example, induce mutations in bacteria or chromosome aberrations in mammalian cells are very carefully evaluated before being used as either flavouring or colouring materials. Chemicals that give negative results in these assays usually undergo a second phase of tests in eukaryotic cells for the induction of gene mutations, and, possibly, for the induction of DNA damage, and for the induction of chromosome damage in rodent bone marrow. Completely negative results in these assays frequently allay concern regarding mutagenic potential with most chemicals. However, additives that are structurally related to known mutagens or carcinogens, and, in particular, chemicals containing a secondary amine structure may be candidates for additional _in vivo_ testing, e.g., germ cell chromosome studies, dominant lethal assays, body fluid mutation tests, etc. Negative results also suggest that the chemical is unlikely to be carcinogenic, but few new food additives are currently released for general use without evidence of the absence of carcinogenic activity in long-term animal studies.

4.5.2.3 Domestic chemical compounds

Cosmetics such as perfumes, hair dyes, sun screen oils, etc., household detergents and cleaning fluids, and a variety of other chemical mixtures are considered under the general heading of domestic chemical compounds. Because of their diverse nature, there have been wide differences in the amount of toxicological information available on these materials and the following examples illustrate the need for caution when considering their safety in domestic use. Several hair dyes of the substituted phenylenediamine type have been shown to be mutagenic in _in vitro_ assays, and some of these have produced cancers in experimental animals. Tris(2,3-dibromopropyl)phosphate is not strictly a domestic chemical but enters the home in the form of a flame retardent in clothing. Widely used to reduce the flammability of children's clothing in particular, the compound was detected as a bacterial mutagen initially, and was eventually shown to be carcinogenic in long-term rodent studies. Fortunately, these are relatively infrequent instances and would have been detected in the base set of two assays now widely used to assess the genotoxicity of new products.

Because these materials are sold for use in an environment where human exposure is to be expected or intended, a complete genotoxicity assessment is usual, and may begin with data from _in vitro_ assays in bacteria and mammalian cells. The sequence of assessment phases described in section 4.3.2.1 is then followed. New chemicals intended for domestic use will normally give unequivocal negative results in tests for gene mutation in both prokaryotic and eukaryotic cells, and for chromosome aberrations in vitro. Where direct contact with the chemical is perceived, data from an in vivo assay for chromosome breakage are usually available. Following the principles developed earlier, positive results in any of these assays may prevent the release of a chemical for domestic use. Evidence from in vivo mutation studies, pharmacokinetic data, or long-term animal studies may, however, remove the concern caused by an isolated positive result in an in vitro assay.

4.5.2.4 Pesticides

Exposure to pesticides may occur in a variety of different ways including exposure of workers during manufacture, exposure during the transport, formulation, or application of pesticides, and exposure to residues in edible crops, soil, and water. Adverse effects on man may result from either the compound itself, its mammalian metabolites, plant and soil metabolites and, possibly, from breakdown products in the environment. Unlike the chemicals described previously as medicinal, food, and domestic chemicals, pesticides are often dispersed widely in the environment and stable materials, such as DDT, may remain as virtually permanent contaminants at minute, though detectable concentrations.

Because of this potential for ubiquity, detailed information on the toxicity, stability, and fate of pesticides in the environment is mandatory in many countries, before they can be registered and released for use. The use of pesticides, however, is virtually indispensible for the successful production of most major crops, and for the control of certain major insect-born diseases of man and domestic animals. This, together with the fact that pesticides are highly biologically-active molecules, requires a fine balance to be set between the benefits accrued by using the pesticide and its possible hazard to man or the environment.

Tests for mutagenicity form only a small part of the overall package of data accumulated before a pesticide is released for use. Short-term tests are usually carried out in parallel with the development of a new pesticide. For example, bacterial mutation data are normally available before the first limited field trials to test the efficacy of candidate compounds are carried out so that safe handling procedures can be formulated for both laboratory and field researchers. The next stage in the development is usually a more extensive field trial on the target crop grown under commercial conditions, and another phase of toxicity testing, including an assay for chromosome aberrations in mammalian

cells, precedes this stage. Unless there is evidence from
other toxicity studies or from chemical structure/pharmaco-
kinetic considerations that the chemical may be genotoxic,
negative results in base set assays frequently allow the
pesticide to proceed through the developmental and evaluation
stages. Where, however, potential genotoxicity is still
suspected, supplementary tests, including assays for gene
mutations or primary DNA damage in eukaryotic cells may be
considered at this time.

The final phase of toxicity testing is carried out after
the development stage is completed and field evaluation has
demonstrated a potentially successful product. These tests
are usually designed to complete the toxicity package required
by most authorities responsible for the licencing of
pesticides for use. Results from a battery of short-term
tests including the bacterial and chromosome assays conducted
during the development phase, an assay for gene mutations in
mammalian cells, and an analysis of metaphase chromosomes of
bone-marrow cells from rodents dosed with the chemical, meet
the requirements of most regulatory authorities. However,
different countries have different requirements, and
additional tests, for example, for aneuploidy or primary DNA
damage, may sometimes be required.

The finding of mutagenic activity in either of the two
initial short-term tests need not necessarily indicate that
development of a pesticide should be abandoned, though this is
often the case. If the potential value of the pesticide
merits further development, it is usually treated as a highly
toxic material and handled accordingly in subsequent field
trials. Additional testing to characterise the mutagenic
activity and to determine its activity in vivo may then be
initiated. An assessment of the hazards associated with a
mutagenic pesticide will depend on data from in vivo studies
(e.g., bone-marrow cytogenetics and either germ-cell
cytogenetics or a dominant lethal assay), the metabolic
profile of the chemical, and data on its stability and rate of
elimination or degradation from the crop and the immediate
environment. A final decision on whether to continue
large-scale development and evaluation of a mutagenic
pesticide may be delayed until data from other biochemical and
toxicological studies, including long-term animal cancer
studies are available.

Pesticides are often supplied and used in a variety of
formulations and in mixtures with other pesticides. It is
usual, therefore, to consider both the pure material and the
specific formulation, when testing pesticides and assessing
the significance of toxicity data.

The assessment of the hazards of residues of pesticides in
plants, soil, and water is usually based on analytical

chemical data. However, some pesticides, e.g., some atrazines, are metabolized by plant enzymes to mutagenic products. Although these metabolites can be analysed chemically, their mutagenic activity can be detected by testing extracts of plants exposed to pesticides in bacterial mutation assays.

Pesticides as a class contain two widely quoted examples of ambiguity between mutagenic activity and carcinogenicity. Dichlorvos (2,2-dichlorovinyl dimethyl phosphate), an organophosphate insecticide, is a confirmed bacterial mutagen. However, results from in vitro mammalian cell assays are either negative or equivocal, and it does not produce mutations in vivo. Comprehensive long-term cancer studies indicate that dichlorvos is not a carcinogen. Pharmacokinetic and other biochemical studies suggest that this compound is efficiently detoxified in animals, so that, in spite of being a bacterial mutagen, it is still marketed as a domestic and agricultural insecticide. The other example is a class of insecticides including DDT and dieldrin known collectively as organochlorine compounds. Both these chemicals induce tumours in liver tissue in mice after prolonged exposure. Both have also been subjected to comprehensive in vivo and in vitro mutagenicity tests, and although isolated positive results appear in the literature, a detailed analysis of the data suggests that these two organochlorines are not genotoxic, i.e., do not cause adverse effects as a direct result of a DNA lesion. The primary carcinogenic growth appears to be confined to rodent liver, and although the potential hazard has been debated at length for many years, the significance of these findings for human health remains unresolved.

Both these examples are given to illustrate the complexity of the extrapolation of in vitro data to animal data to human hazard and serve to emphasise the caution needed in some cases in the assessment of genotoxic hazard from the results of short-term tests.

4.5.2.5 Chemical compounds used in industry

Most industries use chemical compounds in one form or another. The function of the chemical industry itself is to manufacture, from primary sources such as oil, coal, and ore, chemicals that are valuable commodities in everyday life or that are necessary components in the manufacture of other products. The principal raw materials undergo a series of processes to convert them initially to base chemicals (e.g., inorganic compounds such as alkalis and acids, and organic compounds such as olefin and aromatic compounds), then to intermediates and finally to the finished chemical product. These may be consumer products such as solvents, etc., or are

used by other industries in the manufacture of, for example,
paints, adhesives, drugs, and plastics.

The output of the chemical industry is enormous in both
quantity and diversity and the management of safety in the
industry is based on the principle of identifying and
assessing the hazards of exposure to particular chemicals, and
then taking steps to reduce or eliminate human exposure. It
should be accepted that many of the chemicals used in industry
are dangerous to man and a great deal of effort is expended in
ensuring the safety of workers by the introduction of safe
handling procedures, protective clothing, and enclosed
industrial processes.

Exposure to chemicals is possible during manufacture,
during transport of material from one industry to another, and
as a result of environmental contamination. The amount of
toxicity data necessary to provide a sound assessment of the
possible hazard of a chemical is governed primarily by the
extent of human exposure and environmental distribution. For
many of the chemicals used in industry, human exposure is
minimal and data from base set assays are often regarded as
providing sufficient information on the potential mutagenicity
or carcinogenicity of such chemicals to allow the small groups
of workers involved to be protected accordingly. Materials
that are produced in larger volumes and that are transported
in bulk or widely used in other industries may require
additional testing. Bulk products that are non-mutagenic in
the initial battery of tests may need to have these findings
confirmed in, for example, a eukaryotic assay for gene
mutation or primary DNA damage and an in vivo test for
chromosome aberrations, before assessing the genotoxic
hazard. With large-scale chemicals that are shown to be
mutagenic in the base set, the genotoxicity may need to be
further characterised in supplementary in vitro and in vivo
assays. Further testing may involve detailed studies of
mutagenic activity in laboratory animals and long-term cancer
studies may be necessary before the potential hazard can be
fully evaluated and safe working conditions established.

Many chemicals used in industry are volatile and present a
different sort of hazard, for not only can such chemicals
present atmospheric contamination in the workplace, they may
also escape into the surrounding environment. In the modern
chemical industry, the hazards associated with toxic vapours
are well recognised and safe working practices are, in
general, fully implemented, though the toxicity of vapours is
still a real hazard in some cottage industries. When
assessing the mutagenicity of volatile chemicals, it is
important to ensure that the experimental conditions were
appropriate, i.e., in vitro tests require the use of sealed
vessels to eliminate the loss of test material by evaporation,

and, ideally, an inhalation exposure regimen should be used in
in vivo studies.

The manufacture, use, and transport of chemicals used in
industry is strictly regulated by national and international
bodies responsible for industrial and environmental health.
The role of toxicity testing is described in detail in the
guidelines of the appropriate authorities such as the
Organisation for Economic Cooperation and Development (OECD).

5. GLOSSARY

Acentric

chromosomal fragment lacking a centromere

Acrocentric

chromosome with the centromere close to one end of the chromatids

Allele

one of two or more alternate forms of a gene at a specific locus on a particular chromosome

Anaphase

stage of mitosis in which the centromere divides and the chromatids migrate towards poles of the cell

Aneuploidy

addition or loss of one or more chromosomes from the haploid (i.e., meieosis) or diploid (i.e., in mitosis) number, i.e., 2n + 1, 2n - 2, etc.

Autosome

any chromosome other than the sex (i.e., X and Y) chromosomes

Banding

techniques that result in differentially-stained bands along a chromosome, the pattern of banding being characteristic for a particular species and for specific chromosomes; banding techniques are commonly used to identify exchange of material between chromosomes, e.g., translocations

Break

damage to a chromatid or isochromatid involving a discontinuity of the chromosome greater than the width of a chromatid

Bromodeoxyuridine (BrdUrd)   base analogue that is incorporated into DNA in place of thymidine and, using suitable techniques, makes possible the observation of sister chromatid exchanges

Budding and Fission   morphological features of cell division in yeast species

Centriole   cellular component that divides into two prior to mitosis allowing the two daughter centrioles to migrate to opposite ends of the cell forming points of origin of the spindle

Centromere   region at which sister chromatids are held together; also known as the kinetochore, it is the structure by which chromosomes are attached to the spindle; the centromere splits longitudinally at anaphase allowing the chromatids to move to opposite poles

Chromatid   unreplicated chromosome or one half of a complete chromosome with the identical copy being its sister chromatid

Chromatid aberration   structural aberration affecting only one of the two chromatids of a chromosome

Chromosomal aberration   structural aberration affecting both chromatids of a chromosome; also referred to as an isochromatid aberration

Clastogen   a physical or chemical agent that induces chromosome breakage

Cross links   covalent bonds between bases in parallel DNA strands

Deletion	chromatid or isochromatid aberration in which part of a chromosome is missing as a result of a break; the deletion may be from the end of the chromatid, i.e., terminal, or from the middle of the chromatid, i.e., interstitial
Dicentric	a chromosome with two centromeres
Diploid	the normal chromosome number of the somatic cells of most higher organisms; referred to as "2n", where n = the haploid number
DNA	deoxyribonucleic acid
Dominant mutant	term applied to any mutant the effect of which is detectable in the heterozygous condition
Double-strand breaks	rupture of both strands of the DNA double helix at the same site
Endo-reduplication	chromatid alignment is maintained in a cell in which the chromosomes have duplicated but the cell has failed to cleave; a form of polyploidy
Erythroblast	proliferating precurser of red blood cells (erythrocytes)
Extrachromosomal gene	gene carried on an element outside the nucleus, e.g., a mitochondrial gene
Gap	non-staining region of chromatid not larger than the width of the chromatid
Gene conversion	recombination event within a gene producing non-reciprocal product

Giemsa stain	chromosome-staining solution containing the dyes azure, eosin, and methylene blue
Haploid	chromosome number in the gametes; a single set of the chromosomes; referred to as the "n" number of chromosomes
Hemizygous	occurrence of genes in a haploid condition in a normally diploid cell or organism; as on the X-chromosome of _Drosophila_ males
Heterozygote	a zygote derived from the union of gametes, dissimilar in respect of the quality, quantity, or arrangement of genes
Heteroallele	diploid cell carrying two non-identical alleles of a gene
Heterozygote	diploid cells contain two complete sets of chromosomes; the pairs of equivalent chromosomes are called "homologous" and are considered to be structurally identical, at equivalent loci, along the chromsome, alleles of a gene occur which, in homologues, serve the same function; sometimes, the pairs of alleles are not identical and, in such cases, the cell is described as "heterozygous" for the gene at that locus
Hoechst 33258 ®	fluorescent dye used to demonstrate chromosomes in which the DNA has been treated with bromodeoxy-uridine, making observation of sister chromatid exchanges under a fluorescent micro-

Hoechst 33258® (contd). — scope possible; subsequent staining with Giemsa allows observation of sister chromatid exchange under a light microscope

Homoallele — diploid cell carrying two identical alleles of a gene

Homologous — see heterozygote

Homozygote — a zygote derived from the union of gametes identical in respect of the quality, quantity, and arrangement of genes

Hyperdiploidy — aneuploidy in which the chromosome number is greater than 2n

Hypotonic — solution with an ionic strength lower than that of the cell contents; when cells are placed in a hypotonic solution, there is a net uptake of water resulting in swelling of the cell; hypotonic treatment of cells at metaphase improves spreading of chromosomes for microscopic observation

Idiogram (Karyogram) — the arrangement of chromosomes (i.e., from a photograph or drawing) into pairs and groups of pairs, usually in order of decreasing size

Instars — periods in larval development in _Drosophila_; the larvae undergoes two moults so that the larval period consists of three stages: the first, second, and third instars

Intercalation — insertion of a molecule, e.g., adriamycin, between adjacent bases in the DNA molecule

Interchange	exchange of material between two chromatids from different chromosomes
Intrachange	exchange of material between sister chromatids, i.e., on the same chromosome, or exchange within one chromatid
Inversion	chromosome rearrangement in which a region between two breaks has been inverted; "paracentric": the inverted region is within one chromatid arm; "pericentric": the inverted region includes the centromere
Isochromatid aberration	chromosome aberration affecting both chromatids; chromosomal aberration
Karyotype	the chromosome complement of a cell or of a particular species
Lethal gene	a gene the substitution of which, for its normal allele, converts a viable into a non-viable gamete or zygote; may be dominant or recessive
Mating type	in yeasts, mating occurs between strains of opposite mating type, i.e., a and alpha strains in S. cerevisiae and h+ and h- in S. pombe; the genetic event that changes mating type from a to alpha and vice-versa is called a "mating type switch"
Meiosis	cell division in germinal cells resulting in cells with the haploid number of chromosomes
Metacentric	chromosome with the centromere approximately at the

Metacentric (contd).	midpoint; "submetacentric": centromere between the centre and one end of the chromosome
Metaphase	stage of mitosis at which the chromosomes are condensed and aligned on the equator of the spindle
Micronucleus	small fragment of chromosome material visible during interphase outside and separate from the main nucleus; may occur as a result of a chromosome fragment or a whole chromosome that detached from the spindle during mitosis
Minute	very small fragment or minute ring of chromosome material; may occur singly or in pairs
Mis-sense	a mutation producing a gene product with a substituted amino acid
Mitogen	an agent that stimulates resting (interphase) cells to divide and proliferate
Mitotic index	the proportion, usually expressed as a percentage, of dividing cells in a population
Mitosis	stage of the cell cycle at which the chromosomes condense, thus becoming discrete structures when observed microscopically; the chromosomes align on the spindle and then separate into chromatids that migrate to opposite poles of the cell before the cell cleaves to form two daughter cells
Mosaic	a state in which a single individual has cells of two or more different karyotypes

Non-disjunction — failure of chromosomes to separate during mitosis or meiosis resulting in daughter cells with additional and lost chromosomes

Nonsense — mutation producing a messenger RNA molecule with a triplet not coding for an amino acid, e.g., "amber" and "ochre" are nonsense mutations

Normochromatic erythrocytes — mature erythrocytes staining red-yellow with Giemsa stain

Orcein — chromosome-staining solution

Polychromatic erythrocytes — young or immature erythrocytes staining blue-red with Giemsa stain

Polyploidy — cell containing more than the diploid number (2n) of chromosomes in exact multiples of the haploid number (n), e.g., triploid = 3n, tetraploid = 4n, etc.

Recessive mutant — term applied to any mutant the effect of which is detectable in the homozygous or hemizygous condition

Ring — chromosome rearrangement in which fusion of ends of a chromosome results in a ring structure either with (centric) or without (acentric) a centromere

Sex chromosomes — chromosomes that determine the gender of an individual; in mammals, the X chromosome signifies female gender, and the Y chromosome indicates males; diploid cells in normal females are XX and XY in normal males

Single-strand breaks — breakage of only one of the two molecules (strands) in the DNA double helix

Sister chromatid exchange (SCE) — an apparently symmetrical exchange of material between sister chromatids

S-phase — phase in the cell cycle during which normal DNA synthesis occurs

Spermatogenesis — development of the sperm from its precurser cell; successive stages in spermatogenesis are spermatogonia (pre-meiotic), spermatocytes (meiotic stages), spermatids, and spermatazoa (post-meiotic)

Spindle — polymerized tubulin, radiating from the centrioles formed early in mitosis; chromosomes attach to the central point (equator) of the spindle at their centromeres and, subsequently, move along the spindle fibres during anaphase

Spindle poison — agent such as colchicine, colcemid, and vinblastine that prevents tubulin polymerization and thus, chromosome migration, resulting in an accumulation of cells at metaphase; used to arrest cells at metaphase for chromosome examination

SLRL — Sex-linked Recessive Lethals: recessive lethal mutations located on sex chromosomes, i.e., the X-chromosome of _Drosophila_

Suppressor mutation — second site mutation that eliminates the phenotype produced by a previous mutation

Telocentric	chromosome with the centromere at the end of the chromatids
Telophase	stage of mitosis during which the cell cleaves to give two daughter cells
Translocation	isochromatid rearrangement resulting from an exchange of material between two chromosomes
Transposition	transformation of genetic information from one chromosome location to another, e.g., in yeast cells
Vernier reading	location of an object, e.g., a cell, on a microscope slide given as values on two scales (the X- and Y-axis) of the microscopic stage

REFERENCES

ABBONDANDOLO, A. (1977) Prospects for evaluating genetic damage in mammalian cells in culture. Mutat. Res., 42: 279-298.

ABRAHAMSON, S. & LEWIS, E.B. (1971) The detection of mutations in Drosophila melanogaster. In: Hollaender, A., ed. Chemical mutagens: principles and methods for their detection, New York, London, Plenum Press, pp. 461-487.

ADAIR, G.M., CARVER, J.H., & WANDRES, D.L. (1980) Mutagenicity testing in mammalian cells. I. Derivation of a Chinese hamster ovary cell line heterozygous for the adenine phosphoribosyl transferase and thymidine kinase loci. Mutat. Res., 72: 187-205.

ADLER, I.-D. (1970) Cytogenic analysis of Ascites tumour cells in mice in mutation research. In: Vogel, F. & Röhrborn, G., ed. Chemical mutagenesis in mammals and man, Berlin, Heidelberg, New York, Springer-Verlag, pp. 251-259.

ADLER, I.-D. (1974) Comparative cytogenetic study after treatment of mouse spermatogonia with mitomycin C. Mutat. Res., 23: 369-379.

ADLER, I.-D. (1981) Transplacental cytogenetic effects by TEM, mitomycin C, and benzo(a)pyrene. Mutat. Res., 85: 299-300.

ADLER, I.-D. (1982) Male germ cell cytogenetics. In: Hsu, T.C., ed. Cytogenetic assays of environmental mutagens, New York, Allanheld Osmun & Co., pp. 249-276.

ADLER, I.-D. (1985) Cytogenetic tests in mammals. In: Venitt, S. & Parry, J.M., ed. Mutagenicity testing: a practical approach, Oxford, IRL Press, pp. 275-306.

ADLER, I.-D. & BREWEN, J.G. (1982) Effects of chemicals on chromosome aberration production in male and female germ cells. In: Hollaender, A. & de Serres, F.J., ed. Chemical mutagens: principles and methods for their detection, New York, London, Plenum Press, Vol. 7, pp. 1-35.

AHMED, M. & GRANT, W.F. (1972) Cytological effect of the pesticides Phosdrin and Bladex on Tradescantia and Vicia faba. Can. J. Genet. Cytol., 14: 157-165.

ALBANESE, R., TOPHAM, J.C., EVANS, E., CLARE, M.G., & TEASE, C. (1984) Mammalian germ cell cytogenetics. In: Dean, B.J., ed. UKEMS Sub-Committee on Guidelines for Mutagenicity Testing. Part II. Supplementary Tests, Swansea, United Kingdom Environmental Mutagen Society.

AMACHER, D.E. & PAILLET, S.C. (1983) The activation of procarcinogens to mutagens by cultured rat hepatocytes in the L5178Y/TK mutation assay. Mutat. Res., 113: 77-88.

AMACHER, D.E. & TURNER, G.N. (1981) Promutagen activation by rodent-liver post-mitochondrial fractions in the L5178Y/TK cell mutation assay. Mutat. Res., 74: 485-501.

AMACHER, D.E. & TURNER, G.N. (1982a) Mutagenic evaluation of carcinogens and non-carcinogens in the L5178Y/TK assay utilizing post-mitochondrial fractions (S9) from normal rat liver. Mutat. Res., 97: 49-65.

AMACHER, D.E. & TURNER, G.N. (1982b) The effect of liver post-mitochondrial fraction concentration from Arochlor 1254-treated rats on promutagen activation in L5178Y cells. Mutat. Res., 97: 131-137.

AMES, B.N., DURSTEN, W.E., YAMASAKI, E., & LEE, F.W. (1973) Carcinogens are mutagens: a simple test system combining liver homogenates for activation and bacteria for detection. Proc. Natl Acad. Sci. (USA), 70: 2281-2285.

AMES, B.N., MCCANN, J., & YAMASAKI, E. (1975) Methods for detecting carcinogens and mutagens with the Salmonella/ mammalian microsome mutagenicity test. Mutat. Res., 31: 347-364.

ANDERSON, D., BATEMAN, A., & MCGREGOR, D. (1983) Dominant lethal mutation assays. In: Report of the UKEMS Sub-Committee on Guidelines for Mutagenicity Testing, Swansea, United Kingdom Environmental Mutagen Society, pp. 143-164.

ANDRAE, U. & GREIM, H. (1979) Induction of DNA repair replication by hydroxyurea in human lymphoblastoid cells mediated by liver micromes and NADPH. Biochem. biophys. Res. Commun., 87: 50-58.

ASHBY, J., DE SERRES, F.J., DRAPER, M., ISHIDATE, M. Jr, MARGOLIN, B.H, MATTER, B.E., & SHELBY, M.D., ed. (1985) Evaluation of short-term tests for carcinogens. Report of the International Programme on Chemical Safety's Collaborative Study on In vitro Assays, Amsterdam, Oxford, New York, Elsevier Science Publishers (Progress in Mutation Research, Vol. 5).

AUERBACH, C (1962a) Mutation. An introduction to research on mutagenesis. Part 1. Methods, Edinburgh, London, Oliver and Boyd, 176 pp.

AUERBACH, C. (1962b) The production of visible mutations in Drosophila by chloroethyl methylsulfonate (CB 1506). Genet. Res., 3: 461-466.

BAKER, R.M. (1979) Nature and use of ouabain-resistant mutants. In: Hsie, A.W., O'Neill, J.P., & McElheny, V.K., ed. Mammalian cell mutagenesis: the maturation of the test systems, New York, Cold Spring Harbor Laboratory, pp. 237-247 (Banbury Report No. 2).

BAKER, R.M., BRUNETTE, D.M., MANKOVITZ, R., THOMPSON, L.H., WHITMORE, G.F., SIMINOVITCH, L., & TILL, J.E. (1974) Ouabain-resistant mutants of mouse and Chinese hamster cells. Cell, 1: 9-21.

BARTSCH, H., CAMUS, A.-M., & MALAVEILLE, C. (1976) Comparative mutagenicity of N-nitrosamines in a semi-solid and liquid incubation system in the presence of rat or human tissue fractions. Mutat. Res., 37: 149-162.

BARTSCH, H., MALAVEILLE, C., CAMUS, A.-M., MARTEL-PLANCHE, G., BRUN, G., HAUTEFEUILLE, A., SABADIE, N., BARBIN, A., KUROKI, T., DREVON, C., PICOLLI, C., & MONTESANO, R. (1979) Validation and comparative studies on 180 chemicals with S. typhimurium strains and V79 Chinese hamster cells in the presence of various metabolizing systems. Mutat. Res., 76: 1-50.

BARTSCH, H., MALAVEILLE, C., CAMUS, A.-M., MARTEL-PLANCHE, G., BRUN, G., HAUTEFEUILLE, A., SABADIE, N., BARBIN, A., KUROKI, T., DREVPM, C., PICCOLI, S., & MONTESANO, R. (1980) Bacterial and mammalian mutagenicity tests: validation and comparative studies on 180 chemicals. In: Montesano, R., Bartsch, H., & Tomatis, L., ed. Molecular and cellular aspects of carcinogen screening tests, Lyons, International Agency for Research on Cancer, pp. 179-241 (IARC Scientific Publications No. 27).

BARTSCH, H., KUROKI, T., ROBERFROID, M., & MALAVEILLE, C. (1982) Metabolic activation systems in vitro for carcinogen-mutagen screening tests. In: de Serres, F.J. & Hollaender, A., ed. Chemical mutagens, New York, London, Plenum Press, Vol. 7, pp. 95-161.

BATEMAN, A.J. (1958) Mutagenic sensitivity of maturing germ cells in the male mouse. Heredity, 12: 213-232.

BATEMAN, A.J. (1966) Testing chemicals for mutagenicity in a mammal. Nature (Lond.), 210: 205-206.

BATEMAN, A.J. & EPSTEIN, S.S. (1971) Dominant lethal mutations in mammals. In: Hollaender, A., ed. Chemical mutagens: principles and methods for their detection, New York, London, Plenum Press, Vol. 2, pp. 541-568.

BECKER, H.J. (1966) Genetic and variegation mosaics in the eye of Drosophila. Curr. Topics dev. Biol., 1: 155-171.

BENDER, M.A., GRIGGS, H.G., & BEDFORD, J.S. (1974) Mechanisms of chromosomal aberration production. III. Chemicals and ionizing radiation. Mutat. Res., 23: 197-212.

BOLLER, K. & SCHMID, W. (1970) [Chemical mutagenesis in mammals. The bone marrow of the Chinese hamster as an in vivo test system.] Haematologische Befunde nach Behandlung mit Trenimon. Humangenetik, 11: 35-54 (in German).

BOYCE, R.P. & HOWARD-FLANDERS, P. (1964) Release of ultraviolet light-induced thymine dimers and DNA in E. coli K-12. Proc. Natl Acad. Sci. (USA), 51: 293-300.

BOYUM, A. (1968) Isolation of mononuclear cells and granulocytes from human blood. Scand. J. clin. Lab. Invest., 21(Suppl. 97): 77-89.

BRADLEY, M.O., BHUYAN, B., FRANCIS, M.C., LANGENBACH, R., PETERSON, A., & HUMBERMAN, E. (1981) Mutagenesis by chemical agents in V79 Chinese hamster cells: a review and analysis of the literature: a Report of the Gene-tox program. Mutat. Res., 87: 81-142.

BRENNEKE, H. (1937) [Radiation damage to mouse and rat sperm, observed from the early development of the ova.] Strahlentherapie, 60: 214-238 (in German).

BREWEN, J.G. & PRESTON, R.J. (1982) Cytogenic analysis of mammalian oocytes in mutagenicity studies. In: Hsu, T.C., ed. Cytogenic assays of environmental mutagens, New York, Allanheld Osmun & Co., pp. 277-287.

BREWEN, J.G. & STETKA, D.G. (1982) Cytogenetic events in vivo. In: Heddle, J.A., ed. Mutagenicity: new horizons in genetic toxicology, New York, London, Academic Press, pp. 351-384.

BREWEN, J.G., PAYNE, H.S., JONES, K.P., & PRESTON, R.J. (1975) Studies on chemically-induced dominant lethality. I. The cytogenetic basis of MMS-induced dominant lethality in post-meiotic male germ cells. Mutat. Res., 33: 239-250.

BRIDGES, B.A., CLEMMESEN, J., & SUGIMURA, T. (1979) Cigarette smoking - does it carry a genetic risk? Mutat. Res. 65: 71-81 (ICPEMC Publication No. 3).

BRUCE, W.R. & HEDDLE, J.A. (1979) The mutagenic activity of 61 agents as determined by the micronucleus, Salmonella and sperm abnormality assays. Can. J. Genet. Cytol., 21: 319-335.

BRUSICK, D. (1980) Genetic risk estimation. In: Principles of genetic toxicology, New York, London, Plenum Press, pp. 109-135.

BUCKTON, K.E., JACOBS, P.A., COURT BROWN, W.M., & DOLL, R. (1962) A study of the chromsome damage persisting after X-ray therapy for ankylosing spondolitis. Lancet, 2: 676-682.

BURTON, K. (1956) A study of the conditions and the mechanism of the diphenylamine reaction for the colorimetric estimation of DNA. Biochem. J., 62: 315-323.

CALLEN, D.F. & PHILPOT, R.M. (1977) Cytochrome P-450 and the activation of promutagens in Saccharomyces cerevisiae. Mutat. Res., 45: 309-324.

CASKEY, C.T. & KRUSH, G.D. (1979) The HPRT locus. Cell, 16: 1-9.

CLAYSON, D.B. (1981) Carcinogens and carcinogen enhancers. Mutat. Res., 86: 217-229 (ICPEMC Working Paper No 2/3).

CLEAVER, J.E. (1982) DNA damage, DNA repair, and DNA replication in short-term tests for exposure to mutagens. In: Kora, K.C., Douglas, G.R., & Nestmann, E.R., ed. Mutagenesis, human population monitoring, and genetic risk assessment, Amsterdam, Oxford, New York, Elsevier Science Publishers, pp. 111-124 (Progress in Mutation Research, Vol. 3).

CLEAVER, J.E. & THOMAS, G.H. (1981) Measurement of unscheduled synthesis by autoradiography. In: Friedberg, E.C. & Hanawalt, P.C., ed. DNA repair: a laboratory manual of research procedures, New York, Basel, Marcel Dekker, pp. 277-287.

CLIVE, D., FLAMM, W.G., MACHESKI, M.R., & BERNHEIM, N.J. (1972) A mutational assay system using the thymidine kinase locus in mouse lymphoma cells. Mutat. Res., 16: 77-87.

CLIVE, D., JOHNSON, K.O., SPECTOR, J.F.S., BATSON, A.G., & BROWN, M.M.M. (1979) Validation and characterization of the L5178Y TK$^+$/- mouse lymphoma mutagen assay system: Mutat. Res., 59: 61-108.

CLIVE, D., MCCUEN, R., SPECTOR, J.F.S., PIPER, C., & MAVOURIM, K.H. (1983) Report of the Gene-Tox program on L5178Y. Mutat. Res., 115: 225-251.

COLE, J., ARLETT, C.F., LOWE, J., & BRIDGES, B.A. (1982) The mutagenic potency of 1,8-dinitropyrene in cultured mouse lymphoma cells. Mutat. Res., 93: 213-220.

COLE, R.J., TAYLOR, N.A., COLE, J., & ARLETT, C.F. (1979) Transplacental effects of chemical mutagens detected by the micronucleus test. Nature (Lond.), 277: 317-318.

COLE, R.J., TAYLOR, N.A., COLE, J., & ARLETT, C.F. (1981) Short-term tests for transplacentally active carcinogens. I. Micronucleus formation in fetal and maternal mouse erythroblasts. Mutat. Res., 80: 141-157.

COLLINS, A.R.S., SHOR, S.L., & JOHNSON, R.T. (1977) The inhibition of repair in UV-irradiated human cells. Mutat. Res., 42: 413-432.

COMBES, R.D., ANDERSON, D., BROOKS, T.M., NEALE, S., & VENITT, S. (1984) The detection of mutagens in urine, faeces, and body fluids. In: Dean, B.J., ed. UKEMS Subcommittee on Guidelines for Mutagenicity Testing. Part II. Supplementary Tests, Swansea, United Kingdom Environmental Mutagen Society.

CONSTANTIN, M.J. (1976) Mutations for chlorophyll-deficiency in barley: comparative effects off physical and chemical mutagens. In: Gaul, H., ed. Barley genetics. III, Munich, Karl Thiemig.

CONSTANTIN, M.J. & NILAN, R.A. (1982) Chromosome aberrations in barley (Hordeum vulgare): a report of the US Environmental Portection Agency Gene-Tox Program. Mutat. Res., 99: 13-36.

CONSTANTIN, M.J. & OWENS, E.T. (1982) Introduction and perspectives of plant genetic and cytogenetic assays: a report of the US Environmental Protection Agency Gene-Tox Program. Mutat. Res., 99: 1-12.

DARLINGTON, D.C. & LACOUR, L.F. (1976) The handling of chromosomes, 6th ed., London, Allen and Unwin, 201 pp.

DAVIES, P.J., TIPPINS, R.S., & PARRY, J.M. (1978) Cell-cycle variation in the induction of lethality and mitotic recombination after treatment with UV and nitrous acid in the yeast Saccharomyces cerevisiae. Mutat. Res., 51: 327-328.

DEAN, B.J. (1969) Chemically-induced chromosome damage. Lab. Anim., 3: 157-174.

DEAN, B.J. (1985) Summary report on the performance of cytogenetic assays in cultured mammalian cells. In: Ashby, J., de Serres, F.J., Draper, M., Ishidate, M., Jr, Margolin, B., Matter, B., & Shelby, M.D., ed. Evaluation of short-term tests for carcinogens, Amsterdam, Oxford, New York, Elsevier Science Publishers, pp. 69-83 (Progress in Mutation Research, Vol. 5).

DEAN, B.J. & DANFORD, N.D. (1985) Assays for the detection of chemically-induced chromosome damage in cultured mammalian cells. In: Venitt, S. & Parry, J.M., ed. Mutagenicity testing: a practical approach, Oxford, IRL Press, pp. 187-232.

DEAN, B.J. & HODSON-WALKER, G. (1979) An in vitro chromosome assay using cultured rat-liver cells. Mutat. Res., 64: 329-337.

DEAN, B.J., ANDERSON, D., & SRAM, R.J. (1981) Mutagenicity of selected chemicals in the mammalian dominant lethal assay. In: de Serres, F.J. & Shelby, M.D., ed. Comparative chemical mutagenisis, New York, London, Plenum Press, pp. 487-538.

DEAN, B.J., BRIDGES, B.A., KIRKLAND, D.J., PARRY, J.M., & TAYLOR, N.A. (1983) Framework of supplementary testing procedures. In: Dean, B.J., ed. UKEMS Sub-Committee on Guidelines for Mutagenicity Testing. Part 1, Swansea, United Kingdom Environmental Mutagen Society.

DEBAUN, J.R., MILLER, E.C., & MILLER, J.A. (1970) N-hydroxy-2 acetylaminefluorene sulfotransferase: its probable role in carcinogenesis and in protein (methionyl-S-yl) binding in rat liver. Cancer Res., 30: 577-595.

DEMEREC, M., & KAUFMAN, B.P. (1973) Drosophila guide: introduction to the genetics and cytology of Drosophila Melanogaster, Washington DC, Carnegie Institute of Washington, 45 pp.

DE SERRES, F.J. & ASHBY, J., ed. (1981) Evaluation of short-term tests for carcinogens, Amsterdam, Oxford, New York, Elsevier Science Publishers (Progress in Mutation Research, Vol. 1).

DHSS (1981) Guidelines for testing chemicals for mutagenicity, London, Committee on Mutagenicity of Chemicals in Food, Consumer Products, and the Environment, Department of Health and Social Security (Report on Health and Social Subjects No. 24).

DHSS (1982) Guidelines for the testing of chemicals for mutagenicity. V. Genetic and partly-genetic diseases of man: types, frequencies, and mutation rates, London, UK Department of Health and Social Security (Report on Health and Social Subjects No. 24).

DRAPER, M.H. & GRIFFIN, J.P. (1980) Draft guidelines on mutagenicity testing of new drugs issued by the CPMP. A four test screen. Arch. Toxicol., 46: 9-19.

EHLING, U.H. (1977) Dominant lethal mutations in male mice. Arch. Toxicol., 38: 1-11.

EHLING, U.H., CUMMING, R.B., & MALLING, H.V. (1968) Induction of dominant lethal mutations by alkylating agents in male mice. Mutat. Res., 5: 417-428.

EHLING, U.H., MACHEMER, L., BUSELMAIER, W., DYCKA, J., FROHBERG, H., KRATOCHVILOVA, J., LANG, R., LORKE, D., MULLER, D., PEH, J., ROHRBORN, G., ROLL, R., SCHULZE-SCHENCKING, M., & WIEMANN, H. (1978) Standard protocol for the dominant lethal test on male mice. Arch. Toxicol., 39: 173-185.

EHRENBERG, L. (1979) Risk assessment of ethylene oxide and other compounds. In: McElheny, V.K. & Abrahamson, S., ed. Assessing chemical mutagens: the risk to humans, New York, Cold Spring Harbour Laboratories, pp. 157-190 (Banbury Report No. 1).

EPSTEIN, S.S. & SHAFNER, H. (1968) Chemical mutagens in the human environment. Nature (Lond.), 219: 385-387.

EVANS, H.J. (1962) Chromosome aberrations induced by ionizing radiation. Int. Rev. Cytol., 13: 221-321.

EVANS, H.J. (1976) Cytological methods for detecting chemical mutagens. In: Hollaender, A., ed. Chemical mutagens:

principles and methods for their detection, New York, London, Plenum Press, Vol. 4, pp. 1-29.

EVANS, H.J. & O'RIORDAN, M.L. (1975) Human peripheral blood lymphocytes for the analysis of chromosomal aberrations in mutagen tests. Mutat. Res., 31: 135-148.

EVANS, H.J. & SCOTT, D. (1964) Influence of DNA synthesis on the production of chromatid aberrations by X-rays and maleic hydrazide in Vicia faba. Genetics, 49: 17-38.

FAHRIG, R. (1975) Development of host-mediated mutagenicity tests: yeast systems. Recovery of yeast cells out of testes, liver, lung, and peritoneum of rats. Mutat. Res., 31: 381-394.

FAHRIG, R. (1977) The mammalian spot test with mice. Arch. Toxikol., 38: 87-98.

FEDERAL REGISTER (1978) Non-clinical laboratory studies: good laboratory practice regulations. Fed. Reg., 43(247): 59986-60025.

FEDERAL REGISTER (1983) Toxic substances control: good laboratory practice standards. Fed. Reg., 48(230): 53922-53969.

FINK, G.R. & LOWENSTEIN, R. (1971) Simplified method for testing mutagens in Saccharomyces. J. Bacteriol., 100: 1126-1127.

FISCHER, G.A., LEE, S.Y., & CALABRESI, P. (1974) Detection of chemical mutagens using a host-mediated assay (L5178Y) mutagenesis system. Mutat. Res., 26: 501-511.

FOX, M. (1981) Some quantitative aspects of the response of mammalian cells in vitro to induced mutagenesis. In: Marchalonis, J.J. & Hanna, M.G., ed. Cancer Biology Review, New York, Basel, Marcel Decker Inc, Vol. 3, pp. 23-62.

GARCIA-BELLIDO, A., RIPOLL, P., & MORATA, G. (1976) Developmental compartmentalization in the dorsal mesothatic disc of Drosophila. Dev. Biol., 48: 132-147.

GARNER, R.C., MILLER, E.C., MILLER, J.A., GARNER J.V., & HANSON, R.S. (1971) Formation of a factor lethal for S. typhimurium TA 1530 and TA 1531 on incubation of aflatoxin B_1 with rat liver microsomes. Biochem. biophys. Res. Commun., 45: 774.

GENOROSO, W.M. (1969) Chemical induction of dominant lethals in female mice. Genetics, 61: 461-470.

GENOROSO, W.M., CAIN, K.T., KRISHNA, M., & HUFF, S.W. (1979) Genetic lesions induced by chemicals in spermatozoa and spermatids of mice are repaired in the egg. Proc. Natl Acad. Sci. (USA), 76: 435-437.

GOCKE, E., ECKHARDT, K., KING, M.-T., & WILD, D. (1982) Some statistical aspects of spontaneous lethal mutations in Drosophila. Mutat. Res., 104: 239-242.

GRAF, U., JUON, H., KATZ, A.J., FREI, J.J., & WURGLER, G.E. (1983) A pilot study on a new Drosophila spot test. Mutat. Res. Lett., 120: 233-239.

GRAFE, A. & VOLLMAR, J. (1977) Small numbers in mutagenicity tests. Arch. Toxicol., 38: 27-34.

GRANT, W.F. (1982) Chromosome aberration assays in Allum: a report of the US Environmental Protection Agency Gene-Tox Program. Mutat. Res., 99: 273-291.

GRIESEMER, R.A. & CUETO, C., Jr (1980) Toward a classification scheme for degrees of experimental evidence for the carcinogenicity of chemicals for animals. In: Montesano, R., Bartsch, H., & Tomatis, L., ed. Molecular and cellular aspects of carcinogen screening tests, Lyons, International Agency for Research on Cancer, pp. 259-281 (IARC Scientific Publication No. 27).

GUPTA, R.A. & SINGH, B. (1982) Mutagenic responses of five independent genetic loci in CHO cells to a variety of mutagens: development and characteristics of a mutagen screening system based on selection for multiple drug-resistant markers. Mutat. Res., 94: 449-466.

HANAWALT, P.C., COOPER, P.K., GANESAN, A.K., & SMITH, C.A. (1979) DNA repair in bacteria and mammalian cells. Ann. Rev. Biochem., 48: 783-836.

HASEMAN, J.K. & SOARES, E.R. (1976) The distribution of fetal death in control mice and its implications on statistical tests for dominant lethal effects. Mutat. Res., 41: 277-288.

HEDDLE, J. (1973) A rapid in vivo test for chromosomal damage. Mutat. Res., 18: 187-190.

HEDDLE, J.A. & CARRANO, A.V. (1977) The DNA content of micronuclei induced in mouse bone marrow by y-irradiation: evidence that micronuclei arise from acentric chromosomal fragements. Mutat. Res., 44: 63-69

HEDDLE, J.A., BLAKEY, D.H., DUNCAN, A.M.V., GOLDBERG, M.T., NEWMARK, H., WARGOVICH, M.J., & BRUCE, W.R. (1982) Micronuclei and related anomalies as a short-term assay for colon carcinogens. In: Bridges, B.A., Butterworth, B.E., & Weinstein, I.B., ed. Indicators of genotoxic exposure, New York, Cold Spring Harbor Laboratory, pp. 367-375 (Banbury Report No. 13).

HERTWIG, P. (1935) [Sterility phenomena in mice irradiated with X-rays.] Z. indukt. Abstamm. - u. VererbLehre, 70: 517-523 (in German).

HOLSTEIN, N., MCCANN, J., ANGELOSANTO, F.A., & NICHOLS, W.W. (1979) Short-term tests for carcinogens and mutagens. Mutat. Res., 64: 133-226.

HOZIER, J., SAWYER, J., MOORE, M., HOWARD, B., & CLIVE, D. (1981) Cytogenic analysis of the L5187Y TK$^+$1- TK^1 mouse lymphoma mutagenesis assay system. Mutat. Res., 84: 167-181.

HSIE, A.W., O'NEILL, J.P., & MCELHENY, V.K., ed. (1979) Mammalian cell mutagenesis: the maturation of test systems, New York, Cold Spring Harbor Laboratory (Banbury Report No. 2).

HSIE, A.W., CASCIANO, D.A., CROUCH, D.B., KRAHN, D.F., O'NEILL, J.P., & WHITFIELD, B.L. (1981) The use of Chinese hamster ovary cells to quantity specific locus mutation and to determine mutagenicity of chemicals, A report of the Gene-tox program. Mutat. Res., 86: 193-214.

IARC (1979) Chemicals and industrial processes associated with cancer in humans, Lyons, International Agency for Research on Cancer (IARC Monographs Supplement No. 1).

IARC (1980a) Mutagenesis assays with bacteria. In: Long-term and short-term screening assays for carcinogens: a critical appraisal, Lyons, International Agency for Research on Cancer, pp. 85-106 (IARC Monographs on the Evaluation of the Carcinogenic Risk of Chemicals to Humans, Supplement 2).

IARC (1980b) In: Castegnaro, M., Hunt, D.C., Sansone, E.B., Schuller, P.L., Siriwardana, M.G., Telling, G.M., van Egmond, H.P., & Walker, E.A., ed. Laboratory decontamination and destruction of aflatoxins B_1, B_2, G_1, G_2, in laboratory wastes, Lyons, International Agency for Research on Cancer (IARC Scientific Publications No. 37).

ICPEMC (1982) Mutagenesis testing as an approach to carcinogenesis (Committee 2 Report). Mutat. Res., 99: 73-91.

ICPEMC (1983a) Screening strategy for chemicals that are potential germ cell mutagens in mammals (Committee 1 Report). Mutat. Res., 114: 117-117.

ICPEMC (1983b) Regulatory approaches to the control of environmental mutagens and carcinogens (Committee 3 Report). Mutat. Res., 114: 179-216.

ICPEMC (1983c) Estimation of genetic risk and increased incidence of genetic disease due to environmental mutagens (Committee 4 Report). Mutat. Res., 115: 255-291.

ICPEMC (1983d) Estimation of genetic risk and increased incidence due to environmental mutagens (Committee 4 Report). Mutat. Res., 115: 255-291.

IRR, J.D. & SNEE, R.D. (1982) A statistical method for analysis of mouse lymphoma L5178Y cell TK locus forward mutation assay: comparison of results among three laboratories. Mutat. Res., 97: 371-392.

ISCN (1978) Original Article Series 14(8), Basel, S. Karger AG, International System for Human Cytogenetic Nomenclature Birth Defects (Also in: Cytogenet. Cell Genet., 21 309-404).

ISHIDATE, M., Jr (1981) Application of chromosomal aberration tests in vitro to the primary screening for chemicals with carcinogenic and/or genetic hazards. In: Short-terms tests for carcinogens: quo vadis? In: Proceedings of a Symposium held at Montpelier, France (Excerpta Medica), pp. 58-59.

ISHIDATE, M., Jr & ODASHIMA, S. (1977) Chromosome tests with 134 compounds in Chinese hamster cells in vitro: a screening test for chemical carcinogens. Mutat. Res., 48: 337-354.

JENSSEN, D. & RAMEL, C. (1978) Factors affecting the induction of micronuclei at low doses of X-rays, MMS, and dimethylnitrosamine in mouse erhythroblasts. Mutat. Res., 58: 51-65

JOHNSON, R.T. & RAO, P.N. (1970) Mammalian cell fusion: introduction of premature chromosome condensation in interphase myclei. Nature (Lond.), 226: 717-722.

KAPLAN, W.D. & LYON, M.F. (1953) Failure of mercapto-ethylamine to protect against the mutagenic effects of radiation. II. Experiments with mice. Science, 118: 777-778.

KASTENBAUM, M.A. & BOWMAN, K.O. (1970) Tables for determining the statistical significance of mutation frequencies. Mutat. Res., 9: 527-549.

KATZ, A.J. (1978) Design and analysis of experiments on mutagenicity. I. Minimal sample size. Mutat. Res., 50: 301-307.

KELLY, D. & PARRY, J.M. (1983a) Metabolic activation by cytochrome P-450/P-448 in the yeast Saccharomyces cerevisiae. Mutat. Res., 108: 147-158.

KELLY, S.L. & PARRY, J.M. (1983b) The induction of mutation and recombination following UV irradiaion during meiosis in Saccharoymces cerevisiae. Mutat. Res., 108: 109-120.

KIHLMAN, B.A. (1971) Root-tips for studying the effects of chemicals on chromosomes. In: Hollaender, A., ed. Chemical mutagens, New York, London, Plenum Press, Vol. 2, pp. 489-514.

KIHLMAN, B.A. & ANDERSSON, H.C. (1982) Sister chromatid exchanges in plants. In: Wolff, S., ed. Sister chromatid exchange, New York, John Wiley and Sons, pp. 243-265.

KIRKLAND, D.J., GATEHOUSE, D.G., SULLMAN, S.L., VENITT, S., & WATKINS, P. (1984) Bacterial mutation assays with nitrosation products. In: Dean, B.J., ed. UKEMS Sub-Committee on Guidelines for Mutagenicity Testing. Part II. Supplementary Tests, Swansea, United Kingdom Environmental Mutagen Society.

KLASTERSKA, I., NATARAJAN, A.T., & RAMEL, C. (1976) An interpretation of the origin of subchromatid aberrations and chromosome stickiness as a category of chromatid aberrations. Hereditas, 83: 153-162.

KLEWOSKI, E.J., Jr (1978) Detection of mutational damage in fern populations: an in situ bioassay for mutagens in aquatic ecosytems. In: Hollaender, A. & de Serres, F.J., ed. Chemical mutagens, New York, London, Plenum Press, Vol. 5, pp. 77-99.

KLIESCH, U. & ADLER, I.-D. (1983) Chromosome analysis and micronucleus test in mouse bone marrow are not equally sensitive as shown by results with 5 chemical mutagens. Mutat. Res., 113: 340-346.

KLIESCH, U., ROUPOVA, I., & ADLER, I.-D. (1982) Induction of chromosome damage in mouse bone marrow by benzo(a)pyrene. Mutat. Res., 102: 265-273.

KNUDSON, I. (1982) Natural, processed, and artificial mutagens in food: significance and consequences. In: Sorsa, M. & Vainio, H., ed. Mutagens in our environment, New York, Alan R. Liss, pp 315-328.

KRATOCHVILOVA, J. (1978) Evaluation of pre-implantation loss in dominant-lethal assay in the mouse. Mutat. Res., 54: 47-54.

KRUSKAL, W.H. & WALLIS, W.A. (1952) Use of ranks in one-criterion variance analysis. J. Am. Stat. Assoc., 47: 583-621.

KUNZ, B.A., BARCLAY, B.J., & HAYNES, R.H. (1980) A simple, rapid-plate assay for mitotic recombination. Mutat. Res., 73: 215-220.

KUROKI, T., DREVON, C., & MONTESANO, R. (1977) Microsome-mediated mutagenesis in V79 Chinese hamster cells by various nitrosamines. Cancer Res., 37: 1044-1050.

KUROKI, T., MALLAVEILLE, C., DREVON, C., PICCOLI, C., MACLEOD, M., & SELKIRK, J.K. (1979) Critical importance of microsome concentration in mutagenesis assays with V79 Chinese hamster cells. Mutat. Res., 63: 259-272.

KURTEN, S. & OBE, G. (1975) Premature chromosome condensation in the bone marrow of Chinese hamsters after application of bleomycin in vivo. Mutat. Res., 27: 285-294.

LAHDETIE, J. & PARVINEN, M. (1981) Meiotic micronuclei induced by X-rays in early spermatids of the rat. Mutat. Res., 81: 103-105.

LANGENBACH, R., NESNOW, S., TOMPA, A., GINGELL, R., & KUSZYNSKI, C. (1981) Lung and liver cell-mediated mutagenesis systems: specificities in the activation of chemical carcinogens. Carcinogenesis, 2: 852-858.

LATT, S.A., ALLEN, J.W., ROGERS, W.E., & JUERGENS, L.A. (1977) In vitro and in vivo analysis of sister chromatid exchange formation. In: Kilbey, B.J., ed. Handbook of mutagen testing, Amsterdam, Oxford, New York, Elsevier Science Publishers, pp. 275-291.

LATT, S.A., ALLEN, J., BLOOM, S.E., CARRANO, A., FALKE, E., KRAM, D., SCHNEIDERM, E., SCHRECK, R., RICE, R., WHITFIELD, B., & WOLFF, S. (1981) Sister-chromatid exchanges: a report of the Gene-Tox Programme. Mutat. Res., 87: 17-62.

LEE, W.R., ABRAHAMSON, S., VALENCIA, R., VON HALLE, E.S., WURGLER, F.E., & ZIMMERING, S. (1983) The sex-linked recessive lethal test for mutagenesis in Drosophila melanogaster: a report of the US EPA Gene-Tox Program. Mutat. Res., 123: 183-279.

LEIBER, M., SMITH, B., SZAKAL, A., NELSON-REES, W., & TODARO, G. (1976) A continuous tumour-cell line from a human lung carcinoma with properties of type II alveolar epithelial cells. Int. J. Cancer, 17: 62-70.

LEVIN, D.E., HOLLSTEIN, M., CHRISTMAN, M.F., SCHWIERS, E.A., & AMES, B.N. (1982) A new Salmonella tester strain (TA102) with A.T base pairs at the site of mutation detects oxidative mutagens. Proc. Natl Acad. Sci. (USA), 79: 7445-7449.

LINDSLEY, D.L. & GRELL, E.H. (1968) Genetic variations of Drosophila melanogaster, Washington DC, Carnegie Institute of Washington, 472 pp (Publication No. 627).

LONAIT-GALLIGANO, M., LOHMAN, P.H.M., & BERENDS, F. (1983) The validity of the autoradiographic method for detecting DNA repair synthesis in rat hepatocyte primary culture. Mutat. Res., 113: 145-160.

LOPRIENO, N. (1981) Screening of coded carcinogenic non-carcinogenic chemicals by a forward mutation system with the yeast Schizosaccharomyces pombe. In: de Serres, F.J. & Ashby, J., ed. Evaluation of short-term tests for carcinogens, Amsterdam, Oxford, New York, Elsevier Science Publishers (Progress in Mutation Research, Vol. 1).

LOPRIENO, N., ABBONDANDOLO, A., BARALE, R., BARONCELLI, S., BONATTI, S., BRONZETTI, G., CAMMELLINI, A., CORSI, C., CORTI, G., FREZZA, D., LEPORINI, C., MAZZACCARO, A., NIERI, R., ROSELLINI, D., & ROSSI, A.M. (1976) Mutagenicity of industrial compounds: styrene and its possible metabolite styrene oxide. Mutat. Res., 40: 317-324.

LOPRIENO, N., BARALE, R., VON HALLE, E.S., & VON BORSTEL, R.C. (1983) Testing of chemicals for mutagenic activity with Schizosaccharomyces pombe: a report of the US Environmental Protection Agency Gene-Tox Program. Mutat. Res., 115: 215-233.

MA, T.H. (1982a) Tradescantia cytogenetic tests (root-tip mitotis, pollen mitosis, pollen mother-cell meiosis): a report of the US Environmental Protection Agency Gene-Tox Program. Mutat. Res., 99: 293-302.

MA, T.H. (1982b) Vicia cytogenetic test for environmental mutagens: a report of the US Environmental Protection Agency Gene-Tox Program. Mutat. Res., 99: 257-271.

MCCANN, J. & AMES, B.N. (1976) Detection of carcinogens as mutagens in the Salmonella/microsome test: assay of 300 chemicals: discussion. Proc. Natl Acad. Sci. (USA), 73: 950-954.

MCCANN, J.E., CHOI, E., YAMASAKI, E., & AMES, B.N. (1975) Detection of carcinogens as mutagens in the Salmonella/microsome test: assay of 300 chemicals. Proc. Natl Acad. Sci. (USA), 72: 5135-5139.

MACKEY, B.E. & MACGREGOR, J.T. (1979) The micronucleus test: statistical design and analysis. Mutat. Res., 64: 195-204.

MCMAHON, R.E., CLINE, J.C., & THOMPSON, C.Z. (1979) Assay of 855 test chemicals in ten tester strains using a new modification of the Ames test for bacterial mutagens. Cancer Res., 39: 682-693.

MALLING, H.V. (1971) Dimethylnitrosamine: formation of mutagenic compounds by interaction with mouse liver microsomes. Mutat. Res., 13: 425-429.

MANN, H.B. & WHITNEY, D.R. (1947) On a test of whether one of two random variables is stochastically larger than the other. Ann. Math. Stat., 18: 50-60.

MARON, C. & AMES, B.N. (1984) Revised methods for the Salmonella mutagenicity test. In: Kilbey, B.J., Legator, M., Nichols, W., & Ramel, C., ed. Handbook of mutagenicity test procedures, Amsterdam, Oxford, New York, Elsevier Science Publishers, pp. 93-141.

MARON, D., KATZENELLENBOGEN, J., & AMES, B.N. (1981) Comparability of organic solvents with the Salmonella/microsome test. Mutat. Res., 88: 343-350.

MARTIN, C.N., MCDERMID, A.C., & GARNER, R.C. (1978) Testing of known carcinogens and non-carcinogens for their ability to induce unscheduled DNA synthesis in HeLa Cells. Cancer Res., 38: 2621-2627.

MATSUSHIMA, T., TAKAMOTO, Y., SHIVAI, A., & SUGIMURA, T. (1981) Reverse mutation test on H2-coded compounds with the E. coli WP2 system. In: de Serres, F.J. & Ashby, J., ed. Evalutation of short-term tests for carcinogens, Amsterdam, Oxford, New York, Elsevier Science Publishers, pp. 287-395 (Progress in Mutation Research, Vol. 1).

MATTER, B. & SCHMID, W. (1971) Trenimon-induced chromosomal damage in bone-marrow cells of six mammalian species, evaluated by the micronucleus test. Mutat. Res., 12: 417-425.

MEHTA, R.D. & VON BORSTEL, R.C. (1981) Mutagenic activity of 42 encoded compounds in the haploid reversion assay strain XV185-14C. In: de Serres, F.J. & Ashby, J., ed. Evaluation of short-term tests for carcinogens, Amsterdam, Oxford, New York, Elsevier Science Publishers, pp. 414-423 (Progress in Mutation Research, Vol. 1).

MEYER, A.L. (1983) In vitro transformation assays for chemical carcinogens. Mutat. Res., 115: 323-338.

MILLER, E.C. & MILLER, J.A. (1966) Mechanisms of chemical carcinogenesis: nature of proximate carcinogens and interactions with macromolecules. Pharmacol. Rev., 18: 805-838.

MILLER, E.C. & MILLER, J.A. (1971) The mutagenicity of chemical carcinogens: correlations, problems, and interpretation. In: Hollaender, A., ed. Chemical mutagens: principles and methods for their detection, New York, London, Plenum Press, pp. 83-119.

MIRSALIS, J.C. & BUTTERWORTH, B.E. (1980) Detection of unscheduled DNA synthesis in hepatocytes from rats treated with genotoxic agents: an in vivo - in vitro assay for potential carcinogens and mutagens. Carcinogenesis, 1: 621-625.

MITCHELL, A.D., CASCIANO, D.A., MELTZ, M.L., ROBINSON, D.E., SAN, R.H.C., WILLIAMS, G.M., & VON HALLE, E.S. (1983) Unscheduled DNA synthesis tests: a report of the US Environmental Protection Agency Gene-Tox Program. Mutat. Res., 123: 363-410.

MITELMAN, F. (1983) Catalogue of chromosome aberrations in cancer. Cytogenet. cell Genet., 36: Nos. 1-2.

MONTESANO, R., BARTSCH, H., BOYLAND, E., DELLA PORTA, G., FISHBEIN, L., GREISEMER, R.A., SWAN, A.B., & TOMATIS, L., ed. (1979) Handling chemical carcinogens in the laboratory:

problems of safety, Lyons, International Agency for Research on Cancer (IARC Scientific Publications No. 33).

MRC (1981) Guidelines for work with chemical carcinogens in Medical Research Council establishments, London, Medical Research Council.

NCI (1981) Safety standards for research involving chemical carcinogens, National Cancer Institute, US Department of Health, Education and Welfare (US DHEW Publication No. (NIH) 76-900).

NEEL, J.V. & SCHULL, W.J. (1958) Human heredity, Chicago, The University of Chicago Press.

OAKBERG, E.F. (1960) Irradiation damage to animals and its effect on their reproductive capacity. J. dairy Sci., 43(Suppl.): 54-67.

OBE, G., NATARAJAN, A.T., & PALITTI, F. (1982) Role of DNA double-strand breaks in the formation of radiation-induced chromosomal aberrations. In: Natarajan, A.T., Obe, G., & Altmann, H., ed. DNA repair, chromosome alterations and chromatin structure, Amsterdam, Oxford, New York, Elsevier Science Publishers, pp. 1-9 (Progress in Mutation Research, Vol. 4).

OECD (1982a) Good laboratory practice in the testing of chemicals, Paris, Organisation for Economic Cooperation and Development (ISBN 92-64-12367-9).

OECD (1982b) Decision of the Council concerning the minimum premarketing set of data in the assessment of chemicals, Paris, Organisation for Economic Cooperation and Development.

OECD (1984) Data interpretation guides for initial hazard assessment of chemicals (provisional), Paris, Organisation for Economic Cooperation and Development, pp. 58-60.

PARRY, J.M. & PARRY, E.M. (1983) The detection of induced chromosome aneuploidy using strains of the yeast Saccharomyces cerevisiae. In: Kilbey, B.J., ed. Handbook of mutagenicity test procedures, Amsterdam, Oxford, New York, Elsevier Science Publishers, Vol. 2.

PARRY, J.M. & SHARP, D.C. (1981) Induction of mitotic aneuploidy in the yeast strain D6 by 42 coded compounds. In: de Serres, F.J. & Ashby, J., ed. Evaluation of short-term tests for carcinogens, Amsterdam, Oxford, New York, Elsevier

Science Publishers, pp. 468-480 (Progress in Mutation Research, Vol. 1).

PARRY, J.M. & WILCOX, P. (1982) The genetic toxicology in fungi of 4CMB, 4HMB, and BC. Survey of the results of the UKEMS collaborative genotoxicity trial 1981. Mutat. Res., 100: 185-200.

PARRY, J.M. & ZIMMERMANN, F.K. (1976) The detection of monosomic colonies produced by mitotic non-disjunction in the yeast Saccharomyces cerevisiae. Mutat. Res., 36: 49-66.

PARRY, J.M., TWEATS, D.J., & AL-MOSSAWI, M.A.J. (1976) Monitoring the marine environment for mutagens. Nature (Lond.), 264: 538-540.

PARRY, J.M., PARRY, E.M., & BARRETT, J.C. (1980) Tumour promotors induce mitotic aneuploidy in yeast. Nature (Lond.), 294: 263-265.

PERRY, P.E. (1980) Chemical mutagens and sister-chromatid exchange. In: de Serres, F.J. & Hollaender, A., ed. Chemical mutagens: principles and methods for their detection, New York, London, Plenum Press, Vol. 6, pp. 1-39.

PERRY, P.E. & THOMSON, E.J. (1984) Sister-chromatid exchange methodology. In: Kilbey, B.J., et al., ed. Handbook of mutagenicity test procedures, 2nd ed., Amsterdam, Oxford, New York, Elsevier Science Publishers, pp. 495-529.

PERRY, P.E. & WOLFF, S. (1974) New Giemsa method for the differential staining of sister chromatids. Nature (Lond.), 251: 156-158.

PLEWA, M.J. (1982) Specific-locus mutation assays in Zea mays: a report of the US Environmental Protection Agency Gene-Tox Program. Mutat. Res., 99: 317-377.

PMAA (1976) Current good laboratory practices in drug safety evaluation in laboratory animals: guidelines, Washington DC, Pharmaceutical Manufacturers Association of America.

PRESTON, R.J., AU, W., BENDER, M.A., BREWEN, J.G., CARRANO, A.V., HEDDLE, J.A., MCFEE, A.F., WOLFF, S., & WASSOM, J.S. (1981) Mammalian in vivo and in vitro cytogenetic assays: a report of the US EPA's Gene-Tox Program. Mutat. Res., 87: 143-188.

PURCHASE, I.F.H., LONGSTAFF, E., ASHBY, J., STYLES, J.A., ANDERSON, D., LEFEVRE P.A., & WESTWOOD, F.R. (1978) An evaluation of six short-term tests for detecting organic chemical carcinogens. Br. J. Cancer, 37: 873-959.

RASSMUSEN, R.E. & PAINTER, R.B. (1964) Evidence for repair of ultraviolet damaged deoxyribonucleic acid in cultured mammalian cells. Nature (Lond.), 203: 1360-1362.

READ, J. (1959) Radiation biology of Vicia Faba in relation to the general problem, Springfield, Illinois, Charles C. Thomas.

REGAN, J.D. & SETLOW, R.B. (1974) Two forms of repair in the DNA of human cells damaged by chemical carcinogens and mutagens. Cancer Res., 34: 3318-3325.

REVELL, S.H. (1959) The accurate estimation of chromatid breakage and its relevance to a new interpretation of chromatid aberrations induced by ionizing radiation. Proc. Royal Soc. Lond. Ser. B, 150: 563-589.

RINKUS, S.J. & LEGATOR, M.S. (1979) Chemical characterization of 465 known or suspected chemical carcinogens and their correlation with mutagenic activity in the Salmonella typhimurium system. Cancer Res., 39: 3289-3318.

ROWLAND, I.R., RUBERY, E.D., & WALKER, R. (1984) Bacterial assays for mutagens in food. In: Dean, B.J., ed. UKEMS Sub-Committee on Guidelines for Mutagenicity Testing. Part II. Supplementary Tests, Swansea, United Kingdom Environmental Mutagen Society.

RUSSELL, L.B. (1962) Chromosome aberrations in experimental mammals. In: Steinberg, A.G. & Bearn, A.G., ed. Progress in medical genetics, New York, London, Grune and Stratton, Vol. 2, pp. 230-294.

RUSSELL, L.B. (1978) Somatic cells as indicators of germinal mutations in the mouse. Environ. Health Perspect., 24: 113-116.

RUSSELL, L.B. & RUSSELL, W.L. (1956) The sensitivity of different stages in oogenesis to the radiation induction of dominant lethals and other changes in the mouse. In: Mitchell, J.S., Holmes, B.E., & Smith, C.L., ed. Progress in radiobiology, Edinburgh, Oliver and Boyd, pp. 187-192.

RUSSELL, W.L., RUSSELL, L.B., & KIMBALL, A.W. (1954) The relative effectiveness of neutrons from a nuclear detonation and from a cyclotron in inducing dominant lethals in the mouse. Am. Nat., 88: 269-286.

RUSSELL, W.C., NEWMAN, C., & WILLIAMSON, D.H. (1975) A simple cytochemical technique for demonstration of DNA in cells infected with mycoplasmas and viruses. Nature (Lond.), 253: 461-462.

SALAMONE, M., HEDDLE, J., STUART, E., & KATZ, M. (1980) Towards an improved micronucleus test. Studies on 3 model agents mitomycin C, cyclophosphamide, and dimethylbenzanthracene. Mutat. Res., 74: 347-356.

SAN, R.H.C. & STICH, H.F. (1975) DNA repair synthesis of cultured human cells as a rapid bioassay for chemical carcinogens. Int. J. Cancer, 16: 284-291.

SANKARANARAYANAN, K. (1982) Determination and evaluation of genetic risk to humans from exposure to chemicals. In: Bora, K.C., Douglas, G.R., & Nestmann, E.R., ed. Chemical mutagenesis, human population monitoring and genetic risk assessment, Amsterdam, Oxford, New York, Elsevier Science Publishers, pp. 289-321 (Progress in Mutation Research, Vol. 3).

SAVAGE, J.R.K. (1976) Annotation: Classification and relationships of induced chromosomal structural changes. J. med. Genet., 13: 103-122.

SAX, K. (1938) Chromosome aberrations induced by X-rays. Genetics, 23: 494-516.

SCHAEFER, H. (1939) [The fertility of male mice after irradiation with 200r.] Z. mikrosk. -anat. Forsch., 46: 121-152 (in German).

SCHAIRER, L.A., VAN'T HOF, J., HAYES, C.G., BURTON, R.M., & DE SERRES, F.J. (1978) Exploratory monitoring of air pollutants for mutagenic activity with the Tradescantia stamen hair system. Environ. Health Perspect., 27: 51-66.

SCHMID, W. (1976) The micronucleus test for cytogenetic analysis. In: Hollaender, A., ed. Chemical mutagens: principles and methods for their detection, New York, London, Plenum Press, Vol. 4, pp. 31-53.

SCHMID, W., ARAKAKI, D.T., BRESLAU, N.A., & CULBERTSON, H.C. (1971) Chemical mutagenesis. The Chinese hamster bone marrow as an in vivo test system. I. Cytogenetic results on basic aspects of the methodology, obtained with alkylating agents. Humangenetik, 11: 103-118.

SCHMIDT, G. & THANNHAUSER, S. (1945) A method for the determination of deoxyribonucleic acid, ribonmucleic acid, and phosphoproteins in animal tissues. J. Biol. Chem., 161: 83-89.

SCOTT, D., DANFORD, N.D., DEAN, B.J., KIRLAND, D., & RICHARDSON, C.R. (1983) Chromosome aberration assays in mammalian cells in vitro. In: Dean, B.J., ed. Report of the UKEMS Sub-Committee on Guidelines for Mutagenicity Testing, Swansea, United Kingdom Environmental Mutagen Society, pp. 43-64.

SEARLE, A.G. (1975) The specific locus test in the mouse. Mutat. Res., 31: 277-290.

SEARLE, A.G. & BEECHEY, C.V. (1974) Sperm-count, egg-fertilization, and dominant lethality after X-irradiation of mice. Mutat. Res., 22: 63-72.

SETCHELL, B.P. (1970) Testicular blood supply, lymphatic drainage, and secretion of fluid. In: Johnson, A.D., Gomes, W.R., & VanDemark, N.L., ed. The testis, New York, London, Academic Press, Vol. 1, pp. 101-239.

SETLOW, R.B. & CARRIER, W.L. (1964) The disappearance of thymine dimers from DNA: an error correcting mechanism. Proc. Natl Acad. Sci. (USA), 51: 226-231.

SHARP, D.C. & PARRY, J.M. (1981) Induction of mitotic gene conversion by 41 coded compounds using the yeast culture JD1. In: de Serres, F.J. & Ashby, J., ed. Evaluation of short-term tests for carcinogens, Amsterdam, Oxford, New York, Elsevier Science Publishers, pp. 491-501 (Progress in Mutation Research, Vol. 1).

SIMINOVITCH (1976) On the nature of hereditable variation in cultured somatic cells. Cells, 7: 1-11.

SIRIANNI, S.R., FURUKAWA, M., & HUANG, C.C. (1979) Induction of 8-azaguanine and ouabina-resistant mutants by cyclophosphamide and 1-(pyridyl-3)-3, d-dimehytyltriazie in Chinese hamster cells cultured in diffusion chambers in mice. Mutat. Res., 64: 259-267.

SNEDECOR, G.W. & COCHRAN, W.G. (1967) Statistical methods, 6th ed., Ames, Iowa State University Press, pp. 240-242.

SNEE, R.D. & IRR, J.D. (1981) Design of a statistical method for the analysis of mutagenesis at the hypocanthine-guanine phosphoribosyl transferase locus of cultured Chinese hamster ovary cells. Mutat. Res., 85: 77-93.

SOKAL, R.R. & ROHLF, F.J. (1969) Biometry, San Franciso, California, W.H. Freeman and Co.

SORA, S., LUCCHINI, G., & MAGNI, G.E. (1982) Meiotic diploid progeny and meiotic non-disjunction in Saccharomyces cerevisiae. Genetics, 101: 17-33.

STADLER, L.J. (1932) On the genetic nature of induced mutations in plants. Proc. VI Int. Congr. Genet., 1: 274-294.

SULOVKSA, K., LINDEGREN, D., ERIKSSON, G., & EHRENBERG, L. (1969) The mutagenic effect of low concentrations of ethylene oxide in air. Hereditas, 62: 264.

TAN, E.-L. & HSIE, A.W. (1981) Mutagenicity and cytotoxicity of haloethanes as studied in the CHO/HGPRT system. Mutat. Res., 90: 183-191.

TATES, A.D., NEUTEBOOM, I., HOFKER, M. & DEN ENGELSE, L. (1980) A micronucleus technique for detecting clastogenic effects of mutagens/carcinogens (DEN, DMN) in hepatocytes of rats in vivo. Mutat. Res., 74: 11-20.

THOMPSON, L.H. & BAKER, R.M. (1973) Isolation of mutants of cultured mammalian cells. In: Prescott, D.M., ed. Methods in cell biology. IV, New York, London, Academic Press, pp. 209-28.

TJIO, J.H. & WHANG, J. (1965) Direct chromosome preparations of bone marrow cells. In: Yunis, J., ed. Human chromosome methodology, New York, London, Academic Press, pp. 51-56.

TOMKINS, D.J. & GRANT, W.F. (1976) Monitoring natural vegitation for herbicide-induced chromosomal aberrations. Mutat. Res., 36: 73-84.

UNIVERSITY OF BIRMINGHAM (1980) Rules and notes of guidance for the use of chemical carcinogens in the university, Birmingham, The University of Birmingham.

US EPA (1976) An ordering of the NIOSH suspected carcinogens list based only on data contained in the list BP-251851, Washington DC, US Environmental Protection Agency.

US FDA (1979) GLP regulations: management briefings, Washington DC, US Food and Drug Administration (Post-conference Report).

US FDA (1982) GLP regulations: questions and answers, Washington DC, US Food and Drug Administration.

US NAS (1983) Risk assessment in the federal government: managing the process, Washington DC, National Academy of Sciences, National Research Council.

VAN'T HOF, J. & SCHAIRER, L.A. (1982) Tradescantia assay systems for gaseous mutagens: a report of the US Environmental Protection Agency Gene-Tox Program. Mutat. Res., 99: 303-315.

VENITT, S. & CROFTON-SLEIGH, C. (1981) Mutagenicity of 42 coded compounds in a bacterial assay using Escherichia coli and Salmonella typhimurium. In: de Serres, F.J. & Ashby, J., ed. Evaluation of short-term tests for carcinogens, Amsterdam, Oxford, New York, Elsevier Science Publishers, pp. 351-360 (Progress in Mutation Research, Vol. 1)

VENITT, S., FORSTER, R., & LONGSTAFF, E. (1983) Bacterial mutation assays. In: Dean, B.J., ed. Report of the UKEMS Sub-Committee on Guidelines for Mutagenicity Testing. Part 1. Basic Test Battery; Minimal Criteria; Professional Standards; Interpretation; Selection of Supplementary Assays, Swansea, United Kingdom Environmental Mutagen Society, pp. 5-40.

VIG, B.K. (1982) Soybean (Glycine max (L) merrill) as a short-term assay for study of environmental mutagens: a report of the US Environmental Protection Agency Gene-Tox Program. Mutat. Res., 99: 339-347.

VOGEL, E. & NATARAJAN, A.T. (1979) The relation between reaction kinetics and mutagenic action of mono-functional alkylating agents in higher eukaryotic systems. I. Recessive lethal mutations and translocations in Drosophila. Mutat. Res., 62: 51-100.

VOGEL, E., BLIJLEVEN, W.G.H., KLAPWIJK, P.M., & ZIJLSTRA, J.A. (1980) Some current perspectives of the application of Drosophila in the evaluation of carcinogens: In: Williams, G.M., Kroes, R., Waaijen, H.W., & van de Poll, K.W., ed. The predictive value of short-term screening tests, Amsterdam, Oxford, New York, Elsevier Science Publishers, pp. 125-147.

VOGEL, E.W., ZIJLSTRA, J.A., & BLIJLEVEN, W.G.H. (1983) Mutagenic activity of selected aromatic amines and polycyclic hydrocarbons in <u>Drosophila melanogaster</u>. <u>Mutat. Res.</u>, <u>107</u>: 53–77.

VOLLMAR, J. (1977) Statistical problems in mutagenicity tests. <u>Arch. Toxicol.</u>, <u>38</u>: 13–25.

WALTER, E. (1951) [A few nonparametric test procedures.] <u>Mathem. Statist.</u>, <u>3</u>: 31–44 (in German).

WATERS, R., ASHBY, J., BARRETT, R.H., BURLINSON, B., MARTIN, C., & PENMAN, M. (1984) Unscheduled DNA synthesis. In: Dean, B.J., ed. <u>UKEMS Sub-Committee for Guidelines on Mutagenicity Testing. Part II. Supplementary Tests</u>, Swansea, United Kingdom Environmental Mutagen Society.

WATSON, J.D. & CRICK, F.H.C. (1953) Genetical implications of the structure of DNA. <u>Nature (Lond.)</u>, <u>171</u>: 964–967.

WILCOX, P. & PARRY, J.M. (1981) The genetic activity of dinitropyrenes in yeast: unusual dose-response curves for induced mitotic gene conversion. <u>Carcinogenesis</u>, <u>2</u>: 1201–1208.

WILCOX, P., DANFORD, N., & PARRY, J.M. (1982) The genetic activity of dinitropyrenes in eukaryotic cells. In: <u>Mutagens in our environment</u>, New York, Alan R. Liss, pp. 249–258.

WILKIE, D. & GOONESKERA, S. (1980) The yeast mitochondrial system in carcinogen testing. <u>Chem. Ind.</u>, <u>21</u>: 847–850.

WILLIAMS, G.M. (1977) Detection of chemical carcinogens by unscheduled DNA synthesis in rat liver primary cell culture. <u>Cancer Res.</u>, <u>37</u>: 1845–1851.

WILLIAMS, G.M. (1980) Batteries of short-term tests for carcinogen screening. In: Williams, G.M., Kroes, R., Waaijers, H.W., & van de Poll, K.W., ed. <u>The predictive value of short-term screening tests for carcinogenicity evaluation</u>, Amsterdam, Oxford, New York, Elsevier Science Publishers, pp 327–346.

WOLFF, S., ed. (1982) <u>Sister chromatid exchange</u>, New York, John Wiley and Sons.

WURGLER, F.E., GRAF, U., & BERCHTHOLD, W. (1975) Statistical problems connected with the sex-linked recessive lethal test in <u>Drosophila melanogaster</u>. I. The use of the Kastenbaum-Bowman test. <u>Arch. Genet.</u>, <u>48</u>: 158–178.

WURGLER, F.E., SOBELS, F.H., & VOGEL, E. (1977) Drosophila: as assay system for detecting genetic changes. In: Kilbey et al., ed. Handbook of mutagenicity test procedures, Amsterdam, Oxford, New York, Elsevier Science Publishers, pp 335-373.

YAHAGI, T., NAGAO, M., SEINO, Y., MATSUSHIMA, T., SUGIMURA, T., & OKADA, M. (1977) Mutagenicities of N-nitrosamines on Salmonella. Mutat. Res., 48: 121-130.

YAMAMOTO, K. & KIKUCHI, Y. (1980) A comparison of diamaters of micronuclei induced by clastogens and by spindle poisons. Mutat. Res., 71: 127-131.

ZIJLSTRA, J.A. & VOGEL, E.W. (1984) Mutagenicity of 7,12-dimethylbenz(a)anthracene and some aromatic mutagens in Drosophila melanogaster. Mutat. Res., 125: 243-261.

ZIJLSTRA, J.A., VOGEL, E.W., & BREIMER, D.D. (1984) Strain-differences and inducibility of microsomal oxidative enzymes in Drosophila melanogaster flies. Chem.-biol. Interact., 48: 317-338.

ZIMMERMANN, F.K. (1975) Procedures used in the induction of mitotic recombination and mutation in the yeast Saccharomyces cerevisiae. Mutat. Res., 31: 71-86.

ZIMMERMANN, F.K. & SCHEEL, I. (1981) Induction of mitotic gene conversion in strain D7 of Saccharomyces cerevisiae by 42 coded chemicals. In: de Serres, F.J. & Ashby, J., ed. Evaluation of short-term tests for carcinogens, Amsterdam, Oxford, New York, Elsevier Science Publishers, pp. 481-490 (Progress in Mutation Research, Vol. 1).

ZIMMERMANN, F.K., KERN, R., & ROSENBERGER, H. (1975) A yeast strain for the simultaneous detection of induced crossing-over, mitotic gene conversion, and reverse mutation. Mutat. Res., 28: 381-388.

ZIMMERMANN, F.K., MAYER, V.W., & PARRY, J.M. (1982) Genetic toxicology studies using Saccharomyces cerevisiae. J. appl. Toxicol., 2: 1-10.

ZIMMERMANN, F.K., VON BORSTEL, R.C., PARRY, J.M., STIEBERT, D., ZETTERBERG, G., VON HALLE, E.S., BARALE, R., & LOPRIENO, N. (1984) Testing of chemicals for genetic activity with Saccharomyces cerevisiae: report of the US Environmental Protection Agency Gene-Tox Program. Mutat. Res., 133: 199-244.